14D

"Rebuilding trust after an affair is not easy and requires a special kind of support and clear guidance. Scott Haltzman can show you the way. Taking the time to read this book will change your life."

—John Gray, Ph.D., author of *Men Are from Mars, Women Are from Venus*

"Scott Haltzman has done it again—given us a wise, compassionate, and practical guide to the perils and joys of married life. Here he takes on the most shameful and agonizing experience people go through in relationships in a book that helps both the person cheated on and the person who had the affair. Anyone who has gone through this turbulent experience should read it."

—William J. Doherty, Ph.D., professor and director, Minnesota Couples on the Brink Project at the University of Minnesota, and author of *Take Back Your Marriage*

"Scott Haltzman gets down to what's needed: the nitty-gritty details of how to define infidelity, how to end it, and how to recover. The book is so good that it's also a great how-to-avoid-it manual that all married folks should read long before infidelity is even on the horizon."

—Diane Sollee, M.S.W., founder and director, SmartMarriages.com

"In this digital age, more and more couples are finding out where their boundaries are—once they have been crossed. Whether it's friending an old flame on Facebook, sexting someone on Twitter, or flirting online through Skype, many spouses and partners are blindsided and forced to deal with an emotional, online, or real time affair. Thankfully, *The Secrets of Surviving Infidelity* is here. It's a step-by-step survival guide to help your relationship deal with, survive, and overcome the pain of infidelity. If there is 'one last thing' you're willing to do to try to save your relationship from an affair, it should be to read this book!"

—K. Jason and Kelli Krafsky, coauthors of *Facebook and Your Marriage*

"With the infidelity epidemic, every couple needs a survival guide and Scott Haltzman is just the professional to provide it! This common crisis can literally make or break a marriage. Most of those who go on to better relationships do so with expert help. This book is a 'must' for the modern marriage."

—Patricia Love, Ed.D., author of *The Truth about Love*

"For anyone who has felt the pain of infidelity, this compassionate and encouraging book is definitely for you. Based on years of clinical experience and research, Scott Haltzman's step-by-step plan will help you recognize, understand, and then take control of your relationship and your life. One thing is clear—whether you've had an affair or are contemplating one, or you've had a partner who strayed—the knowledge you'll gain from reading this book is invaluable."

— Terri Orbuch Ph.D., relationship expert and author of *Finding Love Again: Six Simple Steps to a New and Happy Relationship*

"As a pro-marriage therapist who works with couples dealing with affairs on a regular basis, I am so pleased to have Scott Haltzman's book available. Couples going through this situation are overwhelmed, confused, and often feel like they are drowning. He has done a wonderful job of explaining in an easy-to-comprehend way all the different types of affairs as well as tools to deal with them. This volume is a wonderful roadmap to assist couples navigating their way back to trust and connection. It's also a great addition to complement therapists doing this type of work."

—Karen H. Sherman, Ph.D., author of *Mindfulness and the Art of Choice: Transform Your Life*

"*The Secrets of Surviving Infidelity* is a very important contribution to this topic. Scott Haltzman is a respected psychiatrist and marriage therapist who has a practical approach to healing from affairs. His book takes a clear stance about avoiding affairs."

—Barry McCarthy, Ph.D., author of *Rekindling Desire: A Step by Step Program to Help Low-Sex and No-Sex Marriages*

"Anyone who has, or is in the profession of helping those who have, or who just wants to know everything about, affairs will benefit from reading this book, and should read it. It is the most comprehensive book on the topic I have seen. I highly recommend it."

—Harville Hendrix, Ph.D., author of
Getting the Love You Want: A Guide for Couples

"This isn't *just* a supremely helpful book on understanding—and recovering from—infidelity. It's a great book on marriage. The honest, warm-hearted, and wise insight Scott Haltzman provides here can bring you hope and much more—a path forward. *This* is the book you are looking for right now."

—Scott Stanley, Ph.D., author of *The Power of Commitment*

"This book provides a wonderfully comprehensive look at all aspects of affairs, including both sophisticated concepts and down-to-earth practical action steps. It is 'must reading' for anyone who wants to survive affairs—or just to improve their marriage."

—Peggy Vaughan, author of *The Monogamy Myth*

"Scott Haltzman's excellent book blends clinical and true-to-life descriptions of the who, what and why of infidelity with profound and personal counsel indispensable for healing the wounds of betrayal. The Secrets of Surviving Infidelity is more than a superb book—it will become your own personal, dynamic counselor navigating you through the pain and confusion of infidelity."

—John Van Epp, Ph.D., author of
How to Avoid Falling in Love with a Jerk

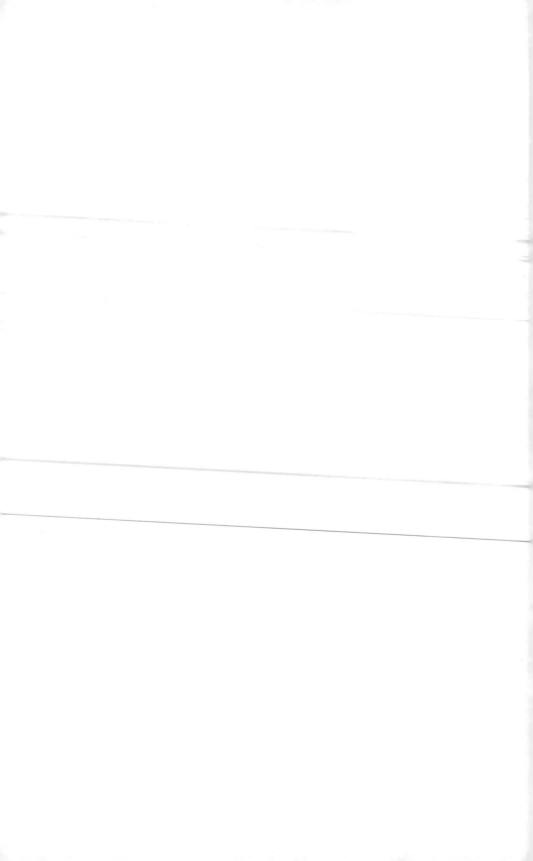

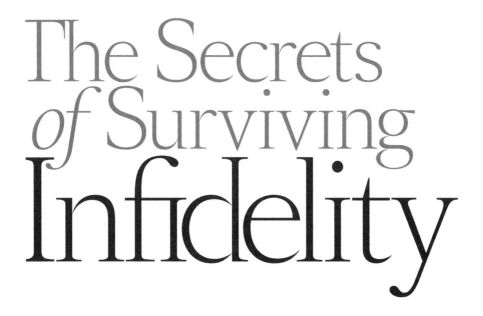

The Secrets of Surviving Infidelity

The Secrets
of Surviving
Infidelity

Scott Haltzman, M.D.

The Johns Hopkins University Press | Baltimore

Note to the Reader: The stories in this book are based on the life experience, clinical work, and research of the author. To protect confidentiality, names and identifying characteristics of clients may have been changed or may represent composite identities of clients. This book describes how people cope with infidelity in general. It was not written about you or your partner or spouse. The services of a competent professional should be obtained whenever medical, legal, or other specific advice is needed.

© 2013 The Johns Hopkins University Press
All rights reserved. Published 2013
Printed in the United States of America on acid-free paper
9 8 7 6 5 4 3 2 1

The Johns Hopkins University Press
2715 North Charles Street
Baltimore, Maryland 21218-4363
www.press.jhu.edu

Library of Congress Cataloguing in Publication Data

Haltzman, Scott, 1960–
    The secrets of surviving infidelity / Scott Haltzman, M.D.
        pages cm
Includes bibliographical references and index.
ISBN 13: 978-1-4214-0941-2 (alk. paper)
ISBN 10: 1-4214-0941-0 (alk. paper)
ISBN 13: 978-1-4214-0942-9 (pbk. : alk. paper)
ISBN 10: 1-4214-0942-9 (pbk. : alk. paper)
[etc]
1. Adultery. 2. Marriage counseling. I. Title.
HQ806.H355 2013
306.73'6—dc23   2012036061

A catalog record for this book is available from the British Library.

Special discounts are available for bulk purchases of this book. For more information, please contact Special Sales at 410-516-6936 or specialsales@press.jhu.edu.

The Johns Hopkins University Press uses environmentally friendly book materials, including recycled text paper that is composed of at least 30 percent post-consumer waste, whenever possible.

For Peggy Vaughan,
a giant in the study of infidelity and a huge-hearted friend

Contents

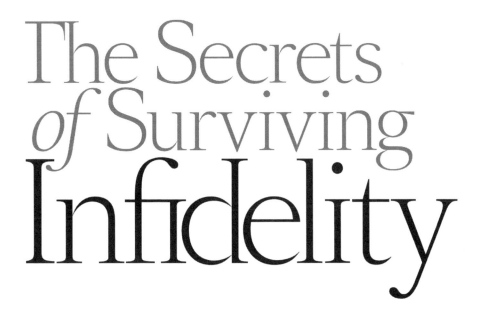

The Secrets of Surviving Infidelity

Prologue

TEN YEARS AGO I was asked to be a guest on the *Today Show* to discuss infidelity in conjunction with the premier of the movie *Unfaithful*. In the movie, Richard Gere and Diane Lane play a happily married couple. After a chance meeting, Lane's character begins a torrid affair with a young and seductive Frenchman played by Olivier Martinez. On the *Today Show*, in the context of this movie, the question Katie Couric asked me was this: "Why do people cheat?"

There was much I could share with the *Today Show* audience about how infidelity affects people and their marriages. For example, of couples who divorce, at least one-third say that infidelity played a role in the dissolution of their marriage. Even among the 50,000 American couples each year who stay together after an affair, returning to a state of stability can take years. Infidelity does not discriminate—it affects people of all races, all religions, and all genders and sexual orientations. It is an intensely emotional topic, and nearly every adult has been affected by it or knows someone who has.

But how could I explain in just a couple of minutes *why* people cheat? Especially considering that Katie Couric, coexpert Helen Fisher, and I all had points we wanted to make. But my appearance on the show clearly struck a nerve, because after the show my website and my e-mail in-box were stuffed full of correspondence. People from all over the world wanted to share their stories and seek advice about the one event that had dramatically altered the course of their marriage: infidelity.

The e-mail messages weren't just from men or women whose partners went outside the marriage for sex; they were also from people who were having affairs and from single people who were having affairs with someone who was married. I heard from children of unfaithful parents, who described how their parent's misbehavior had an impact on them—like 45-year-old Kimberly, who wrote, "My dad, now 81, has lied about his affairs for his entire adult life. The constant lying creates scars that will hurt his kids forever." As I poured through message after message one thing became clear: infidelity doesn't just touch people's lives, it sends shockwaves through their lives. And people wanted to know not just why people cheat but how to survive cheating, whether you are the one cheated on, the one cheating, or the child of a couple whose relationship has been rocked by cheating.

❧ WANTING TO KNOW MORE

As I examined the outpouring of comments following my *Today Show* appearance, it struck me that, although people are fascinated by affairs and long to understand the effect they have on their lives, there's a shroud of secrecy surrounding infidelity that is almost impenetrable. Of course I know that when a person has an affair it's hush-hush—at least until it gets exposed—but that's not the kind of secrecy I'm talking about.

Let me give you an example. When the *Today Show* was preparing to produce the segment about *Unfaithful*, they had asked whether any of my patients would be willing to talk about their experiences on national television. All of my patients politely said, no, thank you. When I sent an announcement over my Internet listserv, there were still no takers. Later I heard from the producers that they had sent out a request to all the viewers of the show and to casting agencies in general, well over half a million people, and still not a single person was willing to be seen on camera and talk about an unfaithful marriage. Think about that: individuals eagerly go on the air to talk about physical and mental diseases, cult involvement, or shattered financial investments. But it's extremely difficult to find someone to publicly discuss a life event that may affect more than one in four Americans.

When I recognized how reluctant people were to step forward and discuss their personal stories, I made a commitment to do everything I could to bring the effects of extramarital relationships out into the open for everyone to see. But before I could do that, I had to understand infidelity better myself.

❧ SEARCHING FOR ANSWERS

I decided to avoid taking the route of great scientists like Jonas Salk or Louis Pasteur—I did *not* go out and have an affair myself. But I asked questions, lots of questions. And much of the information I gathered was through research I conducted on the Internet. At the time, I had been pulling together information to write my first book, *The Secrets of Happily Married Men*, by collecting data about marriage from my website. As part of the writing process, I asked men and women to submit stories and offer solutions on a number of relationship issues. I asked questions such as: "Who's the boss in your relationship?" or "What were your experiences in couple's therapy?" I asked, "What is communication like in your home?" and "How do you deal with conflict?" I also asked about infidelity, because I wanted to know whether and how affairs had impacted people's marriages and whether there were any lessons to be learned from the experience.

I got a broad range of surprising answers. For instance:

When we were dating, I found out my now-husband was running online ads and meeting women. There is a backlash to his past actions. Now, whenever he acts sweet and extra nice to me, I get suspicious and insecure …then I make myself miserable with checking on him, getting internally angry, and mulling over the past. I wish I did trust him and don't know what to do about it.

—Serina, 52, two years into her third marriage

Monogamy is not natural behavior. I have had thoughts and acts of unfaithfulness, yet still have not had sex (of any kind) with anyone but my wife. The passion to express myself and share women's feelings goes far beyond sex. But, without the barrier placed on sexuality by marriage, sex could often be a wonderful expression of feelings.

—Mason, 45, six years into his second marriage

My husband cheated on me. He told me that he made a big mistake, and he's totally ashamed of what he had done. I felt great pain, but time heals. Through this experience we had been more open to each other. We find time to be more intimate and passionate to one another. We talk about our relationship toward each other. More sweet talks and touch, just like when we met each other. Marriage lasts when there's love, communication, friendship, and commitment.

—Nancy, 50, married twenty-one years

Strange as it may seem, my relationship with my wife improves each time I have a short-term affair. Maybe it improves my self-worth. I also compensate by taking extra effort to pay attention.

—Jeremiah, 42, married twelve years

Years of my husband's infidelity has taken its toll on me. Then I had a relationship with a man who taught me the meaning of what a soul mate is. My "soul mate" stayed with *his* wife. So here I am, stuck in Never Never Land, with two men who say they want me but are both incapable of fidelity. Without fidelity, there is no trust, without trust, there is no respect.... I got my heart broken by both my husband and soul mate.

—Kora, 52 years old, married twenty-seven years

I cannot act out any of my fantasies of infidelity because of moral and religious reasons, but I wish there were a way of experiencing such feelings with my husband, as I feel that I have fallen out of love with him. There is nothing as intense as meeting a stranger to fall in love with.

—Rose, 27, married five years

The most important lesson I learned from my patients and from the people who contributed to my Internet research was that when a partner cheats, or is cheated on, it triggers a complex flow of emotions and events that affects everyone involved. These emotions range from rationalization to rage, and when they hit, they hit hard. Even to the point of death. Several of my patients were so devastated when they discovered their spouses' affair that they tried to kill themselves. Relationship issues are the most frequent cause of suicide in the U.S. military.

❧ HELPING OTHERS TO HELP THEMSELVES

This book is about how couples cope when a partner goes outside the committed relationship to seek emotional and physical comfort. Drawing from scientific studies, my research, and my clinical experience, I take you step-by-step through the world of infidelity: How to define it, what to do about it, and how to help you and your mate recover from its shattering effects.

I am not just presenting data or offering advice, though. If you have been personally affected by infidelity, I also want to give you something more difficult to get than facts: I want to give you support and encouragement, while at the same time helping you make sense of something that can seem so senseless. I want to help you feel a little less alone, a little less exhausted, and a little more in control of your life. That's no easy task.

And if you are someone who is straying, or thinking of straying, from your marital vows, I want to help you, too. Few people get involved in an affair without emotional, spiritual, and moral anguish. As I discuss in this book, sometimes it feels as if your desires are beyond your control.

What emotion did you experience that prompted you to pick up this book? Curiosity? Fear? Anger? Depression? Frustration? Relief? I can assure you that whatever you may have felt when choosing this book, and whatever you feel when you read it, there's a good chance that all your feelings are entirely normal.

Let's begin, then, with the basics. Next we'll look at the tricky business of defining what exactly an affair is (you'd be surprised at how controversial the subject is) and how often infidelity touches people's lives.

I

Defining Infidelity

WHEN KAREN CAME TO my office for the first time, she couldn't
hide her torment. She sat down quietly on the couch. Dale came
through the office door a moment later. He sat on the low leather
chair to the left of his wife. We all looked at each other for a moment.
Karen's eyes welled with tears, and Dale looked down.

I knew a little about why this couple was coming to see me. Before
the visit, Karen had called to tell me that she suspected Dale was having an affair. She knew of the work I had done teaching couples how
to have happy marriages and asked whether I dealt with infidelity. I
said yes and then invited Karen and Dale to my office, where they
told me the rest of the story.

Karen works as an interior decorator. She is highly talented and has
been hired by many leading corporations. Dale is a shift supervisor at a
jewelry manufacturing plant who has racked up fifteen years working
at the company and is a respected member of middle management.
Dale is a soft-spoken, even-tempered man with friendly green eyes,
but he's built like a James Bond villain, with muscles bulging out
of his tee shirt. Good-looking and easy-going, Dale was naturally

attractive. Not many women worked with Dale. Unfortunately, it only takes one.

Two days before our appointment, Karen had noticed a late night call placed to an unknown phone number in Dale's cell phone. Karen confronted Dale when he got home from work. At first he said that she was making a big deal over nothing. When pressed, though, he admitted that, yes, "something" was happening with a coworker. But Dale adamantly denied it was an affair. *Something?*

I wasn't there when the initial confrontation took place, but from what the couple told me, it got pretty ugly. Karen was outraged at Dale's behavior and challenged him to justify the potential destruction of a twenty-year marriage and a stable household that included three young girls. Dale, for his part, was furious that Karen accused him of things he had never done or had never meant to do, and he objected to being called the bad guy.

❧ DEFINING YOUR TERMS

Ideally, before two individuals begin to date, and with each advancement in the relationship status, they talk about the parameters of the relationship. At some point in most romances, someone asks, "Are we dating each other exclusively?" If the answer is yes, then that begins a process of developing trust and excluding other people from the relationship. The decision to marry punctuates another formal declaration of "hands off my man/woman." But once two people decide to form a committed relationship, they rarely open up a discussion of what it means to be "unfaithful." There is no one solid definition of infidelity that applies to every situation. Don't conclude, though, that just because a hard and fast definition of an unfaithful act isn't carved in stone, there won't be repercussions whenever a person in a committed relationship makes any physical or deeply emotional contact with a person who is not the life partner.

When one partner accuses the other of an affair, a long course of exploration and explanation opens up. If the confrontation is accompanied by video footage of the spouse performing a sexual act with another person, then there is no room for interpretation. No one yet has come to my office with a video proving adultery. In fact, most people are like Karen and Dale, where the question of cheating is based on some hints of impropriety, with little more to go on. If rules have only been broken in spirit, has there been any infidelity? That depends on how you define infidelity.

The dictionary definition of infidelity mentions "marital disloyalty" and "adultery." The term *adultery* is a legal term that applies when a married person has sexual relations with someone other than his or her spouse. By a dictionary's guidelines, then, infidelity can only take place if marriage has also taken place. While it may be easy for Webster, it's not nearly so clear for the parties involved.

Before we proceed with our discussion of what constitutes infidelity, let's stipulate that it can occur without the institution of marriage. Many of the people I treat in therapy are in committed relationships that don't include an exchange of gold bands. They have decided that they wish to be in a long-term relationship, but they don't, or can't, marry each other. In many states, for instance, gay and lesbian couples aren't allowed to marry. Some people don't marry because they stand to lose money, through tax penalties or loss of alimony or welfare benefits. Thus, when I discuss the different types of infidelity in this book, I include not only married couples, but also couples who have expressed a commitment to monogamy.

When discussing infidelity, it may seem as if any couple who is in a committed relationship should be seen as "married." But it may be more complex than what meets the eye. Many couples who choose not to marry may make a choice to avoid long-term commitment and may be intentionally (or unconsciously) leaving the door open for someone else.

Sexual intercourse: the sine qua non of affairs?

Let's get the most obvious point out of the way from the start: if a person who is married has sexual intercourse with someone other than his or her spouse, that's infidelity. That's pretty clear-cut. But there are shades of gray even here. I'm reminded of an interesting study that asked people about how marital affairs affected them. Men reported that the most upsetting aspect of an affair was the *sexual* contact their wife had. In contrast, the majority of women stated that they were most distraught about their husband's affair if he had formed an *emotional* bond with his paramour.

From the Web: Looking for Sex

My husband doesn't touch me intimately. In the past three years, he would caress my back, shoulder. That's it! He torments me with no sex. Many times I've wanted to go out and just grab some guy and just let loose with all the held-back sex I've built up the past ten years. But for now my sexual urges are still there—constantly needing, hungry, and thirsty for more.

—Margarita, 40, sixteen years into her second marriage

Variations on a sexual theme

One person can betray another in many ways. In the next chapter we look at nonphysical kinds of infidelity, but in this chapter I discuss the physical aspects of infidelity and explore some other ways affairs might be defined. For each of the following physical scenarios, imagine that at least one person is in a committed monogamous relationship, and ask yourself if this could be an affair:

- Two people performing oral sex with each other
- One person performing oral sex or manual sex on the other
- Two people touching each other's genitals without penetration
- One person touching the other's genitals without penetration
- One person touching himself or herself (or performing other sex acts) in front of the other (or in front of a webcam, with the other looking on from a distant site)
- Two people kissing

The answers to these examples, like the example of frank sexual intercourse, may be a pretty obvious yes. But what if these activities are happening with a prostitute during a once-in-a-lifetime business trip? Would that be considered an affair? What if the one person performing manual sex was a masseuse, giving a "relief massage"—also known as a "happy ending"? Would the man on the receiving end of such a massage be considered to be cheating on his wife? (By the way, men aren't the only ones who get erotic massage. As recently as a hundred years ago, physicians treated women's symptoms of anxiety and depression with sexual massage. The vibrator was first invented as a medical tool for the treatment of "hysteria" in women. To this day, some massage parlors offer sexual release for women or men.)

You may be clear that, for you, any of the above examples are, or are not, examples of infidelity. But that doesn't mean that the person you are married to has the same definition of infidelity. After all, despite later revelations that Monica Lewinsky performed sexual activities with a cigar in front of the president, Bill Clinton still maintained: "I did not have sexual relations with that woman."

Infidelity is not about building a relationship. It's about release. For example, I consider it cheating to establish a relationship with another woman just for the sole purpose of having sex. Yet it seems *less* immoral to me to hire an escort. Sex is just sex, but it is important.

—Randolf, 38, married fourteen years

It depends on how you define "sex"

So, does it come down to the definition of sex? And does some form of overt sexual act have to occur for an affair to happen? Consider the following nonsexual physical contacts between a married individual and someone he or she could *possibly* be attracted to, and ask yourself: Do any of these examples violate vows of fidelity?

- Holding hands
- Hugging
- Sitting on another's lap

- Allowing legs to touch each other while being seated side by side
- Resting one hand on the shoulder of someone or allowing that person to do the same
- Playfully pushing or punching another person in the process of joking around or teasing
- Letting fingers linger on each other's fingers when passing an object from one to another

If you're reading this book because you or your partner has had a full-blown sexual relationship with someone outside the marriage, I understand that the scenarios above may seem like trivial offenses in comparison with what you've been through. But countless couples seek counseling because they are experiencing marital fissures over just these kinds of events. For many people, any sort of physical contact with an *attractive person* outside the marriage could be interpreted as cheating.

❧ THE ALLURE OF ANOTHER PERSON

In the previous sentence, I italicized "attractive person." I'd like to take a minute to discuss this phrase, since it's pivotal to understanding the core concerns around marital fidelity and because I use the phrase throughout the book. It would be easy if we could simply say that any married man should avoid any single woman who is younger than him, thin, and looks like Angelina Jolie. Likewise, every woman should avoid all George Clooney look-alikes, especially if he drives a Ferrari and has homes on three continents. And, although for some people such warnings would be spot on, for others they would be insulting. Many men are not attracted to thin women or young women or to any women at all. Women do exist who would not get turned on by someone of George Clooney's looks, style, or steady tone of voice. They may be attracted to older or younger, thinner or more muscular men. Or they may be attracted to women. People define attractiveness on a whole host of characteristics from race to body type to age to personality style. So when I use the phrase "attractive person" I am referring to the *kind of person* who one member of a partnership *could possibly* view as a potential affair mate.

As an example, imagine a husband finds his wife in the act of holding hands with someone. He and his wife know that she is sexually attracted to men, not women, so if his wife were to give another woman a two-handed handshake, and even let it linger as they share a meaningful moment together, this husband wouldn't be the least bit concerned, because that woman holds no attraction for his wife. Likewise, if a wife were to walk into a hospital room while her physician husband was sitting at the bedside of an elderly woman, holding her hand discussing the losses in her life, she would not question his fidelity.

These are the kinds of situations in which there's absolutely no sex appeal, and the issue can be put to rest easily. I'm not saying that every husband or wife knows exactly what kind of person is most attractive to their spouse, but I am saying that you or your mate have some idea of the kind of human beings who are likely to hold an attraction for each of you. And you need to pay attention to these parameters.

Too many people attempt to close the chapter on this discussion without taking a close look at what "attractiveness" means. It's not enough to say, "I'm not interested in my secretary, so why does my wife worry so much?" or to ask, "Why does my husband ask me all these questions about my physical trainer? I'm not tempted by him." *Interest in* is different from *attractiveness to*. If the person is the gender that appeals to you or your partner, falls in the age group that appeals to you or your partner, and has the physical or personality characteristics that appeal to you or your partner, then that person is a potential person of attraction. For one spouse to dismiss the jealousy of the other as absurd simply because there doesn't happen to be an interest does nothing to minimize the fact that that person *is* attractive (at least in the eyes of one of the spouses). In that case, hand holding, hugging, leg or shoulder touching, or even extended handshakes are all cause for concern.

I don't believe that every arm-to-arm brush is an affair. That's ridiculous. But I am saying that any time you cross a physical boundary with an attractive person who is not your mate, there's a lot of room for interpretation and misinterpretation. It's a field of land mines—and you really don't want to go there.

From the Web: Sexual Desires

Recently, I have found myself extremely attracted to a married coworker, who appears to also share the same feelings. I often think about having sex with him . . . just sex!! I don't want to cheat, I love my husband very much, and I would hate myself for hurting him. I think I will try to spice things up in our sex life . . . rather quickly! I'm hoping that my desire for the other man will quickly fade.

❧ WHOSE DEFINITION IS IT, ANYWAY?

One of the problems with books about infidelity—books about anything, for that matter, that try to help people with their specific problems—is that each person searches within its pages to find the answers for his or her specific problem. When I describe general characteristics, limits, and definitions of physicality, in your mind you may feel you don't need any definitions, you know exactly what you or your spouse has done, or might have done, that leads you to pick up this book. So do definitions *really* matter? Yes!

Let's return to Karen and Dale's story. After many weeks of protesting that "nothing happened," Dale finally revealed that he may have gone too far. He admitted to engaging in conversations with his coworker, a single woman ten years his junior named Emily, discussing personal issues related to the quality of his marriage and her past boyfriends. When they visited each other at their workstations, they did touch each other affectionately on the hands, arms, and legs but usually out in the open and not in any overtly sexual manner. He admitted that they talked about having a private get-together and possible sexual liaison in the future but had never actually met each other outside of work.

At this point in the story, particularly if you've ever been involved in infidelity, you might be tempted to blurt out, "Liar!" I get where you're coming from. Like you, I listen to a story like Dale's and my initial thought is, "Of course you did more than touch each other's arms and legs! How do I know you didn't sleep with her?" In chapter 3, we address statistics and how hard it is to determine whether or not infidelity happens, who commits it, and, most important, who admits to it. Many of the stories from people who I see, or the stories posted on my website and sent to me by e-mail, are problematic. After all, in the absence of a Paris Hilton–like video recording or DNA testing of an offspring, it's very difficult to figure out the whole truth, even though the people involved will swear on a stack of Bibles. For the sake of discussion, let's assume that Dale is telling us the whole truth. That some talking and touching happened but nothing sexual ever occurred. Does that meet the criteria for a bona fide affair?

One of the reasons Dale and Karen are dueling over this issue is because they disagree about how to define infidelity. It was very clear in Dale's mind that, although he would've liked to have gone further with Emily, he took the high road and decided not to proceed with any sexual interactions. He felt he prevented an affair. Why should he be demonized for having done the right thing?

In Karen's mind, though, any form of physical touch with another attractive woman represented a breach of their marital vows. But how did Dale know how Karen defined cheating? He figures that since he didn't know his actions represented cheating, he shouldn't be blamed.

Is Dale clueless? That could be, but, based on my clinical assessment, Dale was no dummy. He was a bright, accomplished man who seemed to be an excellent problem solver.

How can Dale be ignorant about something that is obvious to Karen? And how can it be possible that something that is so obvious to *you* can completely bypass your spouse's consciousness? If you have ever had concerns about the way your spouse looks at, touches, lingers around, reaches out to, or in any other way makes physical contact with another person, don't be surprised if he or she thinks you are "making a mountain out of a molehill."

In Dale and Karen's case, we met for several sessions over the next few months. After Dale shared his experience, and he and Karen began the work of healing, one of the first orders of business was for the couple to agree on guidelines for the future. They discussed limiting interactions with people they each might be attracted to. They defined appropriate and inappropriate behaviors, and both agreed that all but perfunctory touch is unacceptable. Rather than feel constricted or bullied by the guidelines, Dale expressed a sense of relief, saying: "Hey, if I know what Karen expects, then it's easier for me to keep myself in line." Like many people in Dale's situation, he looked back at the Emily episode and wished the whole thing had never happened. But now he had an important tool for the future.

❧ A MATTER OF PERCEPTION

Ultimately, smart, well-informed people can still disagree about what form of physical touch violates the marital vows. Consequently, one of the most common stumbling blocks in getting people back on track after an affair is setting clear margins around what kind of extramarital person-to-person contact is acceptable. Karen and Dale were able to get help, and they found a way to solve this problem. In the coming chapters, we will look at how you and your spouse can talk about physical boundaries, clarify your expectations, and come to a mutual understanding to help reduce the risks of infidelity creeping (or creeping back) into your marriage.

Certainly physical connection isn't the only way you can reach out and touch someone. The next chapter explores how emotional relationships can have a huge impact on marriage.

2

What's Emotion Got to Do with It?

UP UNTIL THIS POINT, we have addressed physical touch. We have not nailed down one definition of an affair that would count for everyone; that would be impossible. But it's crystal clear to me that whenever one person engages another in other than perfunctory touching (for example a kiss on the cheek when greeting or a hug at a wake), one must be on the alert for signs of infidelity.

In the sixties, in the midst of the sexual revolution, open marriages, and communal living, people seemed a lot more laid back about sex. During that time, many people believed that being bonded to another person was a spiritual journey. Sexual fidelity was considered a restrictive practice, even a form of involuntary servitude, and committed couples were free to experiment sexually outside of marriage or cohabitation. Have sex with whoever you want, went the philosophy of the time, but be emotionally committed to me. This model didn't work out all that well, and for the most part it died out within a decade. But it raised a concept that hadn't really been discussed before: emotional fidelity.

Here's the crux of the matter: When two people commit themselves to each other they take vows of sexual exclusivity. That's rule number one. But implied in their promise to each other is that they share an exclusive bond spiritually as well as physically. As we saw in the previous chapter, it can be tricky to define physical boundaries—but the challenge is even greater when nonphysical boundaries are crossed.

❧ A SOLDIER'S STORY

Tiffany and Justin are one such couple. Here's what Justin wrote through my Internet message board:

I am recently married, only seven months. I met my wife in the military, so of course she has good relationships with other men. I am currently deployed overseas and have access to our phone records, and I had seen that she had been texting this guy constantly throughout the day and at all hours of the night. Even if we were texting at the same time about sexual things, she would still be texting him between us. I contacted the guy and told him that I am not accusing him and her of anything, but I wanted to inform him that just because my wife and I are currently not around each other, and we may be having fights, we are working on our differences and anyone who comes between me and my family is not going to be happy.

He wrote me back saying that he and my wife went to school together and that they had always been friends who could talk to each other (which she had told me previously). He said he is not the kind of guy to get between a relationship.

I brought it up to her father (where she is currently staying, till I get back) and he told me to leave her alone and stop putting ideas in her head or she will go cheat just because I am blaming her for it.

So I guess my question is: Is it wrong that I am still uncertain of this guy and his intentions with my wife?

Is this cheating? When Justin confronted Tiffany about the issue, she was shocked and offended that he was making such a big deal about it. She insisted that texting a friend throughout the day was not such a big deal. But, as a marital therapist, I have to ask what it is exactly that Tiffany and her school days chum have to talk so much about? For instance, I've been married twenty-five years, my wife and I are crazy about each other, and we love to text (we're *so* twenty-first century!). But if we share even ten texts a day, it's a communication bonanza. So: dozens of texts between Tiffany and her male friend in one day, leading into the wee hours of the night? Maybe they're not romantically involved, but it's clear to me that unless they're texting back and forth to arrange a surprise party for Justin when he returns from the service, they are becoming very intimate with each other.

♣ HOW CLOSE IS TOO CLOSE?

Let's take a look at the word *intimacy*. An "intimate" would be considered a close friend or confidante. And having "intimate relations" is a phrase that my more bashful clients sometimes use to describe sex. When intimacy is used to depict a connection between two individuals, the dictionary defines it as a close, familiar, affectionate, or loving personal relationship. I like to think about it this way: when you dig deep into your heart and come face to face with new insights and perspectives, who do you share your revelations with? The answer to that question tells you who you are intimate with.

There are times when opening up your heart to another person outside of marriage is appropriate. You may choose to discuss your fears, hopes, and frustrations with your parents or your siblings, even if they involve your marriage. Some heterosexual people explore life's unanswered questions with their same-sex barber, hair stylist, or bartender. Even more commonly, straight people will have long conversations with their same-sex friends (or gay people with their opposite-sex friends) in which they delve deeply into all kinds of delicate subjects. Many of my patients share profoundly personal information with me, their therapist. You're not shortchanging your marriage by sharing with another person in any of these cases.

Setting limits

Is there ever a time when unveiling your inner passions to a familiar, attractive (to you), nonprofessional of the opposite sex is okay? Here experts will disagree. But as far as I'm concerned, the bottom line is that any intimate sharing of your life with such a person is a no-no. I'd like to tell you a story that demonstrates that what may be obvious to a marriage expert is not necessarily common sense to a man newly in a committed relationship. And the newly committed man I use as an example is a close friend, Steve, whom I knew through medical school and who met his wife during his residency training.

Before Steve dated his wife, he had a lot of female friends. Some of these women were people he had dated or at least briefly experienced a friends-with-benefits arrangement. But he knew, and they knew, that a long-term emotional commitment just wasn't in the cards. That was cool, they each figured, and they kept in touch. Steve's reasoning for maintaining connections was this: he had invested time and emotions into developing good relationships with these women. They had great personalities and great spirits and had a shared history with him. It didn't seem reasonable to discard all his investments simply because they were no longer dating.

When Steve met his wife-to-be, Sharon, she didn't seem keen on his maintaining female friendships. He was confused at first; after all, he knew that he was committed to Sharon and Sharon only. Why couldn't *she* see that? When they began dating, Sharon and Steve lived and worked about two hours apart. On one particular weekend they weren't able to get together, so Steve invited his most recent past girlfriend to a screening of *Fatal Attraction*. He didn't think there would be any problem, but after Sharon heard about his trip to the cinema, she was not a happy camper.

In retrospect, I believed Steve had missed the irony of the *Fatal Attraction* plot and how it related to him. For those who don't know the movie I can summarize: (1) Happily married man (Michael Douglas) meets new business associate (Glenn Close) when his wife is away. (2) They have what he thinks is a one-night stand. (3) The Glenn Close character becomes obsessed with him and makes his life a living hell. (4) Lots of bad things happen (even to a poor unsuspecting bunny).

Sharon may have trusted that Steve had made his relationship with Sharon paramount, but did Sharon trust the woman he had been dating not to try to seduce him? No. And, did she trust his ability to know when he was being seduced and his ability to resist? No again. I have known Steve more than half my life and to this day I would argue that Sharon had no reason to distrust him, but, hey, let's face it, at the time he was a twenty-six-year-old man raging with testosterone, and it's just possible he might have succumbed to his impulses.

Sharon's instincts told her to beware, and, rather than respect her feelings, Steve chose to go along his merry way. Since he knew she had nothing to worry about, he reasoned that she ought not to worry.

The ABCs of an affair

Steve was wrong. On this occasion, Sharon, with no formal psychiatric training, was dead-on right. Here's why: When Partner A has concerns that Partner B is getting too close to another attractive person, "C," Partner B must respect the feelings of Partner A; Partner A's feelings cannot be ignored or rationalized. One reason is that while Partner B may have no intention whatsoever of getting involved with C, that doesn't mean that C isn't attracted to Partner B. In fact, the very fact that Partner B is in a committed relationship may be a source of attraction to C.

The sixth sense

Many women seem to have a sixth sense for when another woman may be laying the groundwork to move in on her husband. In many of these cases the husband has no clue that this adoring woman has anything but the most honorable motives. Then when his new female friend makes a pass, the husband is shocked and surprised (and, on occasion, he succumbs to it).

There are some biological reasons why a woman may have a better instinct for when her partner is being pursued. Research on the ability to read emotions and nonverbal cues demonstrates that women may have a distinct advantage over men. Simply by looking at pictures of eyes, and no other part of the face, women can determine more accurately than men can whether an individual is feeling anger, desire, boredom, or joy.

And women don't just have special perceptual skills; they also have special skills to attract men. It's often stated that men are the pursuers in relationships. For instance, men often assume that they were the ones who made the first move by asking the woman if she wants a drink, a dance, or anything else he's offering. But close examination of dating rituals shows the opposite: more often than not it's the woman who sends out the nonverbal come hither signs without the guy even knowing. Barely perceptible signals like stroking a bottle, flipping back her hair, touching her chest, or looking down quickly when he looks over are all ways a woman can begin the seduction process. So, if a woman says she suspects that some other gal may be making the move on her man, there's a good chance she's seeing something that he's not. And he'd better pay attention to her instincts.

There may be cases where instincts lead you or your partner to the wrong conclusion, and I talk about that more at the end of the chapter. But too often one partner dismisses another's concerns when the intent of the other man/woman is as plain as day to the rest of the world. If attractive people are in your midst, and you start to share with each other in ways that you believe your spouse would disapprove of, then it's time to ask yourself: Am I starting an emotional affair?

❧ AN EMOTIONAL AFFAIR

If I were to hire a private detective to follow a suspected philanderer around, I would have a pretty clear idea of when a physical connection is happening. His telephoto lens would catch the lurid details:

the handholding, the kissing, or even the more intimate moments. But no camera can capture the emotional part of a relationship, and for many people that becomes the strongest attraction to a person outside of marriage.

From the Web: I Felt Lied to

My husband has broken my heart from the day we wed, I just did not find out about it until later. He pretended to be this respectful person when really he was addicted to relations with plenty of other women. He introduced someone to me as his best friend (a woman) who I always felt weird around and just recently told me they had a sexual relationship right before he started dating me, and the two of them continued flirting through our marriage. And then he had a two-year emotional affair with another woman at work who he had sexual "chats" with. He told her that if things were different he would like to be with her. I feel sick, miserable, and lied to. For the first time in my life I am beginning to wonder if possibly there is such a thing as too much loyalty, if my standing by his side and covering for him is unhealthy codependent behavior. I guess I use the excuse that he has never actually physically cheated since we have been together. What can I say? I was a woman in love who truly believed in the goodness of her man. He has forever changed me, and he has hurt me beyond what I even knew possible.

—Vanna, 29, married five years

Shared feelings

Not every intimacy becomes an emotional affair, but every emotional affair begins with intimacy. Emotional infidelity is defined as the growth of a strong psychological bond between two individuals who are not in a committed relationship when one (or both) of them is married to someone else. If neither of these individuals were hitched, they might just be considered to share a really strong friendship. But because at least one of them is in a committed relationship, this is much, much more than a friendship. An emotional affair includes the following: sharing intimate secrets, seeking to spend time alone with each other, and withholding information about the relationship with one's spouse. When important things happen in the life of people in this situation, rather than wanting to notify their mates, their first thought is to tell their intimate friend.

There is debate among experts about whether emotional affairs really exist, but here's my take on it: Before you got married, you promised that you would not give yourself sexually to anyone but him or her. But you also implicitly promised that you would only give yourself *emotionally* to that one person. When your thoughts are with another person even as you are in your life partner's arms, that's a problem. You're withholding an important portion of yourself from your mate and giving that part to a person who is not part of your family. In other words, you're *cheating* your partner out of something that's rightfully his or hers.

There's no question about it: maintaining a healthy marriage takes a lot of emotional work. Consider the tremendous amount of energy required every day to keep a marriage thriving (or surviving), and compare that with how much time and effort goes into being with, thinking about, obsessing over, connecting with, and daydreaming over the *other* person. I think you'll agree that any person who distracts that degree of attention away from the marriage is a potential threat to the stability of that marriage.

From the Web: Stealing Attention

I see any time that my husband spends paying attention to a woman other than me as stealing. He is stealing time that he could be focusing on our marriage or relationship. I don't care if its two minutes or five hours, that's enough time to make dinner reservations or arrange for a babysitter.

Shared experiences

All kinds of stuff in life require you to spend time with another person, everything from getting a project done at work to picking up dry cleaning. Clearly, simply being in the same room with someone doesn't mean you're on the fast track to destroying your wedding vows. Consider, though, the comments of Laurie Puhn, lawyer and marriage mediator, in her book *Fight Less, Love More*: "The core of emotional intimacy is shared experience." That very succinct definition sums up why one spouse feels cheated when the other repeatedly shares rich and meaningful experiences with someone else. If, as Forrest Gump's mother would say, "Life is like a box of chocolates," then emotional infidelity is like someone reaching into your mate's box and stealing some chocolates. Rightfully, those chocolates, good or bad, are yours—and nobody else's—to ingest with your life partner.

Not everyone agrees with my point of view, here. One of the contributors to my website, Lydia, wrote:

It seems to me that when people get married, every single decision is made on the basis of how it will impact the marriage. Is there no time when you are acting only for yourself? Why is it so harmful for a person to have a special experience of his or her own? If I get married I fully expect to keep seeing my friends, to go to movies, to go to restaurants, to do sports, to develop hobbies alone or without my partner every once in a while. Some people would consider any of these activities some kind of threat to the marriage, but it's fairly sensible to assume that having a bit of your own life can actually keep your marriage interesting because of the constant infusion of stimulation from outside. So, what's the difference between these activities and sharing my body for one night with another person?

It's not always "just sex," sometimes you learn things about yourself and people from making love that are really important.

Notice the phrase, "If I get married"? Lydia is single. Earlier in her correspondence with me, she admitted to a brief relationship with a married man "who is very much in love with his partner of several years." I wonder if, once Lydia does get married, she will realize that marriage itself builds a closeness and vibrant emotional life that affairs can neither produce nor sustain.

Willard Harley, author of *His Needs, Her Needs,* has helped thousands of couples heal from marital problems. One of the ways he does it is by recommending that couples spend at least fifteen hours a week, each week, with only each other, doing recreational activities, being affectionate, talking, or having sex. And by "only each other," he means *without kids*. Many couples balk at his advice, noting that they can barely get even two minutes—let alone two hours—a day of alone time together. But here's how Dr. Harley justifies his recommendations: the average amount of time a person spends with someone they're having an affair with is, you guessed it, fifteen hours a week! Hidden in this statistic is a deeper point, that spending time—time talking, time laughing, time just hanging out—with another person builds a sense of emotional closeness. So if you're out and about with an attractive person, even if you are not in physical contact with that person, you may be at risk for having an emotional affair. And if you're hanging with Lydia, it could become downright sexual.

❧ CROSSING A BOUNDARY

One of the biggest misconceptions about infidelity is that it usually involves a person (or two people) who is on the prowl for sex and gets a special buzz out of the idea of sneaking around while getting it. Yes, it is true that there are thrill seekers who just can't settle into the routine of married life. Studies show, for example, that extroverts are more likely to have affairs than are introverts. And, yes, there are some people who are driven by incredibly high levels of testosterone and incredibly low self-control. (We'll talk more about why people have affairs in chapter 4.) But most affairs take place between two people who had *absolutely no intention* of cheating. These two people meet, befriend each other, find each other interesting, and then, well, one thing leads to another. In some cases, it can take just one night for it to happen. In some instances, it can be between neighbors who have known each other for years. In all these cases, if you were to ask what led up to it, most people would honestly say, "We never intended for an affair to happen." That's why two people in committed relationships must be very careful about the kinds of interactions they have with people outside of their home. Even if there's no intention of an affair, there's a risk.

Ethan and Marie came to see me for help. Ethan had one physical affair and one emotional affair, and the couple, who had already separated once, was at risk for splitting again. I began to see Ethan, a successful architect, alone in my office, where we talked about some of the issues dealt with in this chapter. Ethan caught on quickly and made great strides to getting back on track. But Ethan had a problem; he was an extrovert with good looks and a great personality. Several of the female clients who met Ethan in the waiting room commented on what a nice guy he was, and even my secretary commented on his sex appeal. Most single guys would kill to be in Ethan's shoes, but as far as Ethan was concerned, women's attraction to him was a curse, because every time a woman locks eyes on him, Marie fumes.

Marie isn't alone in her anguish. Many people are just naturally appealing to others. For example, pharmaceutical salespeople are chosen by multibillion-dollar firms for their physical attractiveness and people skills. It's not hard to imagine that many of their spouses are frustrated by how easily people are drawn to their mate. Whether an individual is naturally attracted to a married person, or the attraction grows over time, no person can afford to be ignorant of the impact that such emotional connections make on a life partner. The real question is: Once a married person begins to feel a connection to another person, what happens next?

From the Web: Building Walls

A relationship is like a brick wall. When you are in the dating stage, you are building that wall, and once you are married that wall should be strong and solid. If you lie, cheat, or have any type of affair, that damages the trust you have for one another, and when you do that, it puts cracks in the wall you are trying to build. In this case, the wall can only stand so strong, last so long, with the cracks and punctures before it breaks and falls apart. I feel as though a relationship is the same way. You can only try to build on something broken for so long, and the fact of the matter is you cannot have a strong relationship with someone when the relationship was built on lies.

Lee, the family friend

The key to safeguarding your relationship from falling prey to an affair is to make certain that any attractive individual whom you have as a friend is a *friend of the marriage* (or committed relationship). Let's say that you like spending time with Lee, and Lee lives one block over. Lee is the same sex as your mate. Lee is about your age, in good physical shape, and not unappealing to the eyes. Lee is outgoing and has a great sense of humor. Can Lee become your friend? Yes, but Lee can't become your private friend. In order to be able to enjoy a warm friendship with Lee, Lee has to be part of the family. Your first meetings with Lee should exclusively be in the company of your mate. If your partner thinks Lee is a laugh-and-a-half and values Lee's company, then Lee is a friend of the marriage. While most times you, Lee, and your partner buddy up, you may occasionally spend time with Lee alone—*but only with the blessings of your partner.* Let's say your mate hates Louisiana music, but Lee and you really like zydeco. Lee and you decide to go to a local Cajun concert, and while there, you text your spouse a few times, and fill in all the details when you get back. When you talk to Lee on the phone, you tell your partner about it. When your partner picks up the phone, Lee doesn't immediately ask for you but chats for a while with your spouse. That's a friend, and a friend of the family. Someone like Lee could well be a friend for life.

The slippery slope

In substance abuse circles, there is a phenomenon referred to as the "slippery slope," in which one is able, at each step, to assert absolute sobriety . . . until it's too late. One of my patients with a fifteen-year history of alcohol abuse, including severe liver damage, made the decision to get sober after an emergency room visit where her blood alcohol level was five times the legal limit. After two weeks of drying out, she left the detox center swearing off alcohol for life. She moved out on her substance-abusing boyfriend, began to go to Alcoholics Anonymous (AA) meetings, and reconnected with her sober daughter and granddaughter.

On our follow-up visit one week later she told me she still wasn't drinking, but she had moved back in with her boyfriend. On the next visit, she told me that she stopped visiting her family because her daughter didn't approve of her decision to stay with the boyfriend: "But I still don't drink." Two weeks later, she told me that she still had not had a drink, but she had stopped going to her AA meetings because she felt people there were "too judgmental."

From my point of view, this capable and bright woman completed detox on firm footing, but after that she made decisions that pulled her downward. With each choice she justified what she did; initially the fact that she had not relapsed proved her right. I think you know where I'm going with this story: what do you think happened to this woman a few weeks after she stopped her meetings, cut off her healthy social support systems, and moved back in with her substance abusing boyfriend? Bingo! She's back to drinking.

Emotional relationships can also succumb to the slippery slope effect; the biggest risk is that they can lead to physical affairs. Any of the small steps away from absolute devotion to your mate risk putting you on the wrong course. The unanticipated results could destroy your marriage.

From the Web: We Only Ever Shook Hands

I have had thoughts and acts of unfaithfulness yet still have not had sex (of any kind) with anyone but my wife. The first woman I had thoughts about I came to love deeply. For two years we talked, had lunches, and shared all, even our sexual selves. We only ever shook hands, to avoid physical stimulation. She married another and moved away. The second, we found each other while I was on a business trip. We dined and went to shows. We kissed and cuddled. At first I declined sex, but the next time we met she declined. We still have contact, e-mail and telephone. We both express a great desire for a complete feeling. I do believe that if we meet again, sex is inevitable (so, no plans to meet). My love and devotion to my wife are intact.

—Moises, 45, six years into his second marriage

Setting parameters

In some cases it's not clear whether someone is a friend of the relationship. In those cases, each partner must seek the opinion of the other. If there is someone of the opposite sex (or, of the same sex if you are so attracted) who you enjoy spending time with, you need to take a close look at what that friendship is like. Here are six guidelines to help figure out whether someone of the opposite sex can be considered a true friend.

1. *If it feels wrong, maybe it is wrong.* Your mate must feel comfortable around this person. He or she doesn't necessarily have to feel spiritually bonded to your friend, but there should be a sense of feeling at ease about your spending time with him or her. Your new friend must be willing to form a connection with your partner and your family. Not just as a pro forma act so he or she can spend time with you, but out of genuine interest in being a part of your family.

2. *Keep no secrets.* Your friend should not ask you to keep any secrets from your mate. You should not share any secrets with your friend that you have not told your mate or would be unwilling to have your friend share with your mate. Never be in a position to say to your friend: "I'm telling you this because my partner wouldn't understand" or otherwise hint that your friend appreciates you in ways that your mate does not. Also, any and all contact with your friend should be in full knowledge of your partner. If you find yourself meeting with your friend by accident somewhere, you should immediately contact your partner to say: "Just ran into our friend . . ."

3. *Elevate your mate.* Under no circumstances should your friendship include discussions about your mate's faults in anything but the most general terms. Pointing out that a plant died because "LeMar doesn't have a green thumb" is acceptable; commenting that the garbage cans are outside because "LeMar never does his chores around the house" is not. Likewise, your friend should not use your relationship to talk about faults in his or her partner, if there is one.

4. *Avoid sexual situations.* You should not talk about any sexual issues with your friend. It's fine to discuss how outraged you are with

the local politician who got caught soliciting a prostitute, but any discussion about your sexual preferences or experiences is strictly off limits. Avoid situations that foster physical intimacy, such as long dinners in dim lighting, sitting in hot tubs without spouses around, or slow dancing to Harry Connick Jr. You may not feel any romantic inclination toward your friend before doing these things, but the right situation can breed new interest. You should never engage in excessive drinking or any illegal drug use with this friend, as sharing "sins" together develops false intimacy, and substance abuse lowers inhibitions.

5. *Share your time.* You should not develop habits of exclusively having alone time with your friend. It's critical that your family periodically be included in get-togethers. Be very cautious about regular rituals that you and your friend have. It's okay to say "Every year we run the Boston Marathon together," but not "Every morning we have coffee together," unless you have complete buy-in from your partner.

6. *Pay attention to your inner voice.* If you begin to feel a romantic attraction to the other person, or if this person begins to express one to you, you must immediately break off all contact with that person.

Learning by example

Many "attractive" married individuals are able to have great relationships with other attractive married people. These couples do things together as foursomes. They camp together, vacation together, watch Super Bowls together, and sit up all hours of the night talking together. They may stop in and check up on each other once in a while, but each spouse tells their mate and all are comfortable with the arrangement. These individuals may conclude a phone conversation with a platonic "Love you!" In these friendships, all of the six guidelines have been followed. These are friends of the marriage.

Contrast this arrangement to that of Dan, a patient of mine, a young college professor who had met a Spanish girl, Maria, through a foreign exchange program when they both were teenagers. A year after Dan had married Liza, Maria visited from Madrid. She was cordial to Liza but not warm. In private she told Dan that she was there to see him, not his wife or newborn child. She denied having any romantic interest, and Dan believed her. But Liza was not happy with Maria and was convinced that she was no friend of their marriage. Liza asked Dan to cut off ties with Maria, which he did. It was the right thing to do.

❧ TIME TO TAKE ACTION

But is it fair?

Dan didn't break off his relationship with Maria quite as willingly as Liza had hoped he would. Still early in his marriage, Dan didn't exactly know the difference between "my friend" and "a friend of the marriage," and cutting off ties with this particular friend did not happen without some real soul-searching on his part.

When Liza first said that she and Dan should have nothing further to do with Maria, Dan protested vigorously. He had known Maria long before he knew Liza and had invested many years in a friendship with her. In fact, not only was he friendly with Maria but so were his parents and siblings. Sure, Dan had kissed Maria a few times when he was sixteen, but they were both kids then. Dan acknowledged that Maria was rude to Liza, but he knew Maria's personality, so he made accommodations for it.

Liza saw it differently. Although Dan was no longer romantically interested in her, Maria was still unmarried and obviously had maintained an interest in him. So Liza, using her highly attuned intuitive abilities, smelled trouble whereas Dan smelled nothing but fresh air. Dan thought Liza was way off base. He felt like her accusations were an assault on his integrity (though they were really an attack on Maria's integrity). He felt like Liza didn't trust him (though she really didn't trust Maria). And he felt that she didn't have faith in their marital vows (though what she knew was that faith alone doesn't keep marriages together). In Dan's words, "Liza was asking me to give up a friendship that I had cultivated for a decade because of her neurotic concerns."

After years of working with married couples and researching infidelity, I can say definitively: Dan was wrong. And situations similar to Dan's and Liza's may well be a sore point for you if you are reading this book. You may have been asked to remove yourself from an innocent friendship, and you may be feeling resentful about your mate's request.

When it's time to end friendships

We can see this very thing happening in the message from Justin in the beginning of this chapter. While Justin is overseas in the military, his wife is maintaining a texting relationship with an old male friend. Justin questions whether this is appropriate, and Tiffany tells him he's overreacting. Then, on top of it, Tiffany's parents tell Justin to butt out! In my opinion, Justin isn't overreacting; he's making good sense. The interactions between his wife and her old school chum are inappropriate. She should honor Justin's concerns and drop this friendship. Now. By doing so, not only does she demonstrate respect for Justin, but also she validates and protects the marital bond.

Throw out that "little black book"

Justin and Tiffany's case seems clear to me, but in many relationships preventing infidelity will sometimes result in collateral damage. On occasion, a friendship that seems perfectly innocent will need to be ended in order for you or your spouse to rest easy. Admittedly there are cases of what psychiatrists call "pathological jealousy," in which one partner sees a threat in every interaction their partner has with everyone he or she ever meets. If you or your partner is in this situation, then I recommend you get the opinion of a trained mental health practitioner who can help you sort out what's reasonable and what's overboard. But assuming that neither you nor your partner has this condition, you can still expect that you will still need to shorten your friends list on Facebook.

For those who are serious about committing to their marriage, making it last for life, and not doing anything to jeopardize it, avoiding the formation of close friendships with members of the opposite sex isn't that difficult. It's a small sacrifice to pay for maintaining a loving and successful marriage.

You may feel resentful or angry about needing to let go of friendships you've developed over the years. But, here's the choice you have to make: you can either make your friend happy or make your spouse happy. Who did you make a lifetime commitment to? Which decision do you think will make you happier in the long run?

From the Web: "I could easily have fallen"

I have learned to keep my distance from male coworkers and, yet, through required daily interaction, have felt pangs of attraction going both ways. I have extremely high self-esteem, thankfully, as well as a strong sense of right and wrong. Had I not, I could easily have "fallen" when I felt the pangs of attraction. Instead, I took the high road, and backed off from the interactions. Not that difficult.

❧ HELPING YOUR PARTNER SEE THE LIGHT

I'm a big believer in having people take control of their own lives, so if you are crossing the friendship frontier without your partner's approval, you have to rethink your priorities. There's a good chance that if you are reading this chapter you're doing just fine, however, and it's your partner's behavior that's a concern to you.

I received this question from Bebe on my DrScott.com forum that encapsulates the difficulties in finding a definition of emotional infidelity that both partners can understand:

My husband has an overwhelming need to have female relationships and I don't know what else to do short of ending our six-year relationship. From the very beginning I knew that our marriage was going to be challenging specifically because his pick up line was that he already had enough female friends and that he was looking for something more. I accepted his forwardness and tried to build a friendship with him while we dated. Early on he explained to me that his best friend was a woman he had known eight years. I wasn't completely happy about it at the time. We've since then gotten married and have one daughter.

My problem is based on the nature of his work; he always wants to be with the young ladies from his office. Even the ones who have left their jobs with him continue to call him and vice versa.

I have no patience for cheating. In the past, he's made some poor decisions to be too chummy with females from the office, and now I don't trust him. I don't know if we're going to make it through this. At every turn there is some new female friend calling or text messaging. I am a jealous person by nature, but I try not to project that on to him. To make matters worse. My husband is the Social Suzy of his office and a Chatty Cathy. Those two combinations don't go very well. I don't want to give up but I can't do the female friendship thing.

I respond:

You've invested a lot in the marriage, and, as you say, you knew who he was before you married him (I'll bet he's reminded you of this frequently when you lodge complaints). But I understand why you'd be worried and hurt. If he wants the marriage to work, then ask him to read *Not Just Friends* by Shirley Glass.

Knowledge is power, and if he knows the best way to be a husband (that includes not having close women friends who aren't also friends of yours) then he needs to hear it from an authority. (No, sorry, you don't qualify as an authority.)

Bebe answers:

Thank you for the book recommendation. My husband definitely has mommy issues that play a major role in how he relates to women. He just needs to have and be around women. He gets giddy and thrives at the idea of women sitting around gossiping. He has virtually no deep male bonds and has expressed to me that he would like to pursue them but finds himself unable to nurture friendships with his male friends. I talked with him this morning, after looking at our phone records and seeing that he made and received very lengthy (thirty minutes or more) daytime phone calls on his cell from two women in particular on a frequent basis. I know both of the women fairly well, but I still expressed to him that I don't think it's appropriate and that these women should respect our relationship and not call a married man so frequently.

He flew off the handle and said that I was trying to control his friendships and that he wasn't doing anything wrong. After about two hours of arguing, I finally made my position clear and gave him an ultimatum, which basically said that if he wanted to continue to be married to me, I was not accepting, acknowledging, or condoning any new female friendships unless they were mutual. I told him that he had not earned my trust based on past errors of judgments to even have casual friendships and that he could take it or leave it. I stood my ground, waited a couple of hours, and then he relented. Now I have to see if he will actually follow through. I need to know if there is a simpler way of getting him to realize the error of his ways.

I respond:

The problem with issuing an ultimatum is that if your husband doesn't understand the rationale, then you come across as being illogical or unreasonable. If I gave my wife an ultimatum of either she learns to fire a rifle or I'm leaving the home, she'd think I was nuts, and she would still not pick up a gun. If I turned on the news and showed her that a buffalo stampede was heading toward our house, she'd understand why I wanted her to learn this new skill.

It may be common sense to you that your husband cease and desist or get out, but he may not appreciate your reasoning. If he does stop interacting with women, he'll do so resentfully, and it will take a long time to heal that rift. It took me years of study in the field to understand this issue; don't expect him to understand it because you tell him what his change in behavior must be.

Your best bet is to get him to appreciate and accept the concepts underlying *why* you are looking for a behavior change. That should be the only challenge or ultimatum right now—for him to take the time to understand where you are coming from. As I pointed out, sometimes that requires an outside "expert," since he may not accept your point of view as valid, that's why reading a book on the subject may be a good step.

Surviving infidelity ultimately requires knowing what infidelity is. You and your partner probably didn't begin the marriage with the same understanding of what "having an affair" means, but I think you're finding that having a meeting of the minds is an important task moving forward. That's why, if being the victim of emotional infidelity is central to why you're reading this book, then this is one chapter you will want your partner to read.

When sorting out who to connect with, and who to avoid, you might be wondering whether infidelity is really that much of a risk to you or your mate. In the next chapter, we'll look at the data about how frequently affairs happen and how often people will really admit to the truth.

3

What the Numbers Tell Us

IN READING ABOUT POTENTIAL marital transgressions in chapters 1 and 2, it would be easy to reach the conclusion that just about everyone cheats by someone's definition. Indeed, the situations described in the previous chapters do happen to most couples at some time. In many cases they happen early in a relationship as couples adjust to the challenges of being one of a pair, but they never cross the line into unfaithfulness. These experiences highlight how effortlessly infidelity can intrude into happy, healthy marriages and how easy it is to transition from happy and healthy to miserable and dysfunctional. Exactly how many relationships does infidelity affect? Let's take a look.

From the Web: "My wife announced she had an affair"
I have been married for seven years, and, although they haven't been perfect, they have been quite good. Six days ago, my wife announced she had an affair with her boss. I'm devastated and confused.

I'm trying to take it moment by moment at this point, but am not sure what I am going to do. After finding out how often they met and that half of the time they were in our bed and unprotected, I was convinced I wanted a divorce. Over this past weekend, I started to soften but have been faced with a cold reaction from her—she has not shed a tear and today became defensive, telling me what I have done wrong over the last few months.

Things are a mess right now. I've lost thirteen pounds this week and missed a day of work because I was dizzy and nauseous because I forgot to eat for four days. But, what concerns me the most is now I go from staying to divorcing in my mind about fifty times a day.

✥ LIES, DAMNED LIES, AND STATISTICS

Mark Twain once said, "There are three kinds of lies: lies, damned lies, and statistics." The first time I heard this line, I thought it meant how people can bend statistics around to suit their needs. But when I began to research the question of infidelity statistics, this quote kept popping into my mind. Because when it comes to figuring out whether people are cheating on each other, it's almost impossible to know. After all, when researchers arrive at a home, poised with pen and paper in hand asking about marital affairs, who's going to run to the door and say, "Me! Me!"? Nobody! So, if you want to find out about marital stats, you'd better be ready for some big lies.

I'm reminded of the clever way marriage expert Michele Weiner-Davis begins a training exercise for clinicians. She points out how common affairs are, and then, as if to highlight her point, asks the audience, "Raise your hand if you've had an affair."In the moment that follows comes a wave of uncomfortable silence, before everyone finally breaks out in laughter. And all the while not a single person's hand shoots into the air. Michele's point is brought home by a study done by University of Colorado researchers, who discovered that when people were given an anonymous questionnaire, their rate of admitted infidelity went up sixfold.

As we've discussed in the previous two chapters, it's not exactly clear what a researcher means when she asks, "Have you ever had an affair?" Although most studies limit the definition to "sex with someone outside of marriage," that doesn't include all those potentially marriage-busting acts (such as texting a man at 2 a.m. or spending your paycheck at a strip bar) that many couples see as betrayals. Published studies also ignore people who are not married but are in committed relationships. For example, in states that don't allow gay marriage, how does a researcher define a same-sex partner who strays?

From the Web: "Not perfect anymore"

My first husband was the perfect gentleman. Well, not perfect anymore, because I found out he cheated on me, made a woman pregnant, had a son with her, and in the two years I stayed with him he kept it a secret.

—Ashanta, 25, now in her second marriage

♣ WHOSE STATISTIC IS IT, ANYWAY?

Does it really matter what the statistics say? After all, if you're reading this book, then there's a good chance that infidelity (or a near affair) has already affected you. For quite a few people, knowing how frequently others are affected by affairs is irrelevant. *If it happened to me,* they reason, *then it happened to 100 percent of everyone who matters.*

Many people find the statistics helpful, though. The maxim "misery loves company" takes form in the relief that some victims of infidelity feel knowing that they are not alone. One of the most frequent emotions felt by a betrayed spouse is total isolation. Some of my patients whose spouses cheated tell me they feel like a failure. Some were so convinced that their family and neighbors would judge them harshly that they isolated themselves: they stopped going to social events, and they refused to answer the phone. Statistics can be very important to these people; when they see how many other people are similarly impacted, they don't feel so alone.

Lila, for example, told me that she had just found out about an affair that her husband had had more than fifteen years earlier. Her life had completely shut down when she found out. Already a thin woman, she had lost more than twenty pounds in the few months since her husband had confessed. She was lost. At the end of our first session, I told her about some supportive websites and recommended some literature. By the time she returned for our second session, she had already begun to rally. Her appetite picked up, and she began to involve herself in life again. She explained, "I had felt so cut off from everyone before. Now I know that this has happened to so many other people and that people can survive it. I'm sure I can survive it, too." Two years later, she is still going strong.

Sometimes unfaithful spouses (or the single person they are cheating with) will take comfort in the statistics for all the wrong reasons. "See!" they say, while pointing to the charts and graphs, "Affairs happen all the time. Why are you giving me such grief?" But, while data about infidelity highlight the vulnerability that everyone has, they can still be valuable for people who are considering an extramarital tryst. The married man who is in seventh heaven because he believes he has found his (non-wife) soul mate may feel like the odds of such a thing happening are one-in-a-million. He may feel compelled to follow his heart and end his marriage in order to start with the "right" person. Knowing that the odds are actually closer to one-in-three is a bit humbling and may bring him down to earth a little.

From the Web: "Hot boss"

I seem to be attracted to my boss more every day. Besides the fact that he's *hot*, he also has a great personality and sense of humor. I feel I can connect with him like I would with one of my female friends. Like soul mates. We are both fortyish and married with children.

I don't know if he is attracted to me or not, I just feel overwhelmingly drawn to him, like a soul mate kind of thing. It sounds silly, but I have never felt this kind of connection with anyone of the opposite sex before. I have felt close to my female friends in this way, but never a male. It's like we unconsciously connect. I know I need to redirect my attention, but if we are ever put in the situation, I don't know if I can refuse.

♣ THE ENVELOPE, PLEASE!

How frequent are affairs? As I said, it depends on how you define affairs, who you ask, and how they interpret the numbers. Among experts, there is no consensus on this issue. One of the most widely acknowledged statistics is this: about 1.5 percent of people will have an affair for each year of marriage. Not so bad, you might think. But that's only *per year*. In other words, after ten years the rates go up to 15 percent, and after twenty years, 30 percent of married people have had an affair.

This statistic highlights a paradox. Most people assume that the longer a couple has been married, the greater the strength of the union. That's supported by the data that show that an awful lot of spouses end their marriage within the first few years. But, the longer you're married, the more time you have for things to happen: the more likely you are to win the lottery, get in a car accident, or see an albino deer munching on your vegetable garden. That's why some researchers at the University of Chicago have come up with what appear to be puzzling findings. While they show pretty consistently that every year, 10 percent of spouses admit to cheating (12 percent of husbands, 7 percent of wives), people who are over the age of 60 actually have the highest rates of infidelity over a lifetime. For those of you who think of this population as the ones who populate the "Help I've Fallen and I Can't Get Up" commercials, remember that, at the time of the study, 60-year-olds would have included Mick Jagger, Eric Clapton, Tina Turner, and Carly Simon. I'm not saying that any of these rock stars had affairs, but I am painting a picture for you of what life was like when people who are now sixty were coming of age. They lived in some wild times!

These data tell us that among the 60-plus crowd, 28 percent of all men and 15 percent of all women have had at least one affair. These studies don't make clear which homes have had both husband and wife having affairs, and which homes were affected by only one person's infidelity, so the total number of marriages that are affected ranges from 28 to 43 percent.

I did warn you that not all research is created equal. When Shere Hite, author of the *Hite Report,* published data on affairs, she concluded that 70 percent of American women who were married for more than five years had broken their marriage vows at least once. I know that sounds outrageous; even I think that's out of bounds. But I recall a very unscientific discussion with one of my mentors from medical school, who maintained a very successful Park Avenue practice, and he claimed that every single one of his patients had had an affair at one time or another.

The take-home message from all this research is loud and clear. Affairs are not rare. Remember that exercise you did in your assemblies in high school (whether the subject was bullying, drug addiction, or STDs)? You know the one—where the speaker at the podium tells you to look to your right, then look to your left, and that either you or one of the people you are looking at will be affected by _____ (fill in the blank with bullying, drug addiction, STDs, or whatever else the speaker is trying to convince you to avoid). Well, I'm that speaker. Look to the house on the left of you, look to the house on the right. Research tells us that your home or one of these other two homes will have someone who is affected by infidelity.

If that home is yours, it doesn't mean you have to lose hope or lose face. The next chapters examine the causes of infidelity. Understanding "why?" is the first step toward finding ways to recover from its devastating effects.

4

Why People Cheat

PEOPLE DESIRE CONNECTION. PEOPLE want to feel special. People want to feel love. People have a hunger for sex. People like the feelings that happen inside their bodies when they feel a romantic attraction.

And that's why people get married.

You probably thought I was writing about why people have affairs, and, truth be told, I was writing about that as well. The qualities that draw you to your husband-to-be or wife-to-be are very much like the forces that pull you into another intimate relationship.

Consider the Web contribution of 40-year-old Gwyneth:

I became seriously involved with a man (also married with children) during my second and current marriage. He was the ultimate knight on a white horse. Very good looking, body-builder, romantic, poetic, the whole nine yards. He told me his sob story about his miserable marriage, and I fell for it and him. At the time, I felt very undesirable and unloved by my husband. No, I'm not blaming my behavior on the way my husband treated me, but the door wouldn't have been open for someone else to swoop in if I had truly felt that I was the most important person in my husband's life.

My husband and I did discuss my involvement with the other man, and it almost destroyed him and our relationship. And the other man almost destroyed me.

I have learned the hard way that an affair is *not* the answer. My husband and I managed to pull through, and we now treat each other as if tomorrow might not come. We've been together a total of eighteen years and are still friends, still have earth-shattering sex, and yes we still fuss every now and then. But hey, we're normal.

Gwyneth's short story lays out all the elements that lead to affairs: a desire to connect with another person, a wish to feel needed and important, and the allure of sexual arousal. What's more, Gwyneth says she felt "undesirable and unloved" by her husband. (Notice that this statement says as much about her *feeling* toward her husband as it does about his actual *actions*. There's an important difference between how one person acts and how the other perceives it. This is a big issue, and we'll return to it in chapter 9.) No one aspect of human passion can alone explain why Gwyneth, or anyone, will have an affair. In my opinion there is no good reason for infidelity, period. But, to paraphrase the ubiquitous bumper sticker: *Affairs Happen*. And if there's any hope of fixing the problem in your life, then it's worth figuring out why.

So let's start at the beginning. In the following section of this chapter, I'll be talking about heterosexual relationships, because that's what best helps to explain many (although not all) features of animal and human bonding.

☘ THE LAW OF ATTRACTION

Understanding animal sexual behavior can unlock mysteries from mating pandas to keeping bees. Organic farmers, for instance, to whom pesticides are off limits, use knowledge of sex hormones to kill off Japanese beetles during infestations. They employ an ingenious contraption called a "beetle trap." The trap is constructed of a bright yellow hard plastic plate suspended above a plastic bag. The plate, infused with a combination of a flower and sex hormone scent, attracts beetles. Driven wild by the smell, the beetles charge headlong toward the plate. They then crash into the hard plastic and fall into the bag, where they can't get out again. This simple contraption can take thousands of beetles out of commission in a matter of days. I can't say how much of what drives those beetles into the bag has to do with floral scent and how much has to do with the allure of the pheromones. The way I see it, the beetles probably tell themselves that there is a good nectar meal ahead and some good sex to follow.

We don't need beetle traps to prove that animals are driven to all kinds of behavior for the sole purpose of reproduction. All kinds of stupid human tricks are done solely for the opportunity to have sex. While most people wouldn't run full speed into a plastic wall, most of us know people who have done things almost as outrageous for a chance to hook up with someone.

In reality, it takes more than pheromones and a dinner out for two humans to feel a sexual attraction. But don't underestimate the power of hormones when it comes to the lure of the opposite sex. The primary hormones involved in sexual attraction are *testosterone* and *estrogen*. Testosterone, found in greater amounts in men, increases sex drive and triggers assertive behavior. A man's testosterone level doesn't change significantly from day to day. In healthy men it's usually high, and most men are ready for sex just about all of the time.

Women respond to reproductive urges also, and, believe it or not, they are also driven by testosterone. About halfway through a woman's monthly cycle, her estrogen levels begin to rise, and, as she reaches the peak of her fertility, testosterone levels also peak. In this brief time, women are more likely to be attracted to men. Scientists have shown that a man's repulsive sweat-soaked tee shirt will actually smell good to a woman during (and only during) these fertile times. Women report a 24 percent increase in sexual activity during their fertile phase.

❧ FROM HORMONES TO NEUROCHEMICALS

A hormone is defined as a chemical that, while produced in one gland of the body, moves through the blood to have an effect on a different part of the body. Testosterone, for example, is produced in the testicles of men, and estrogen is produced in the ovaries of women. Yet, because they travel throughout the body, these chemicals have profound effects on the entire body, from how your muscles develop, to whether you develop acne, to how frequently you think about sex. Often these two hormones can be responsible for a couple meeting and having a strong desire to rip each other's clothes off. From this strong sex drive comes a feeling, if only for an instant, that the proud owners of these hormones may be "in love."

Love at first sight may exist, but as far as scientists are concerned, this desire to jump in the sack with a suddenly irresistible and incredibly attractive individual is lust—plain and simple. Don't pooh-pooh lust; after all, this hormone-driven craving for sex is responsible for the propagation of our species for the past hundred millennia or so. Playwright and novelist W. Somerset Maugham, who is often quoted as saying, "Love is a dirty trick," puts it plainly: "There is no object to life. To nature nothing matters but the continuation of the species." But, while the hormonal need to reproduce can partly explain why people are attracted to each other in the first place, it doesn't explain why they *stay* attracted to each other. For that, we need to take a close look at brain chemicals that affect our emotional balance. These chemicals are called *neurotransmitters*, and they are considerably different from hormones.

Hormones are produced in glands in the body, but neurochemicals are produced in little chemical factories stored in the tips of our brain's nerve cells. Unlike hormones, which travel through the body to have their effects, neurochemicals don't move through blood to do their job—they stay within the brain and conduct business where they are manufactured.

Deeply imbedded in the most primitive parts of the brain is a series of brain nerve cells (called *neurons*) that send off chemical signals that unconsciously tell the body what to do and what to feel. Automatic behaviors, such as breathing or temperature regulation, even the need to sleep, are directed by this part of the brain, called the *brainstem*. The brainstem transmits information to the conscious parts of the *cerebral cortex* (the more sophisticated part of the brain) so that your basic needs are made clear to you. For instance, if you become dehydrated, you may suddenly have a craving for a glass of water. You are not consciously aware that your electrolytes are out of whack; you just know that you want to drink fluids. These neurochemicals are not unique to humans. In fact, as complicated as the human brain is, these same chemicals are found deep in roots of our neurological system in parts of the brain that exist in animals much lower on the evolutionary scale.

Scientists have logged millions of hours trying to sort through the effects of different neurotransmitters, not only to figure out how we feel but also how we plan, react, relax, and store memories. When it comes to romance, research has narrowed in on three specific neurotransmitters: *norepinephrine*, *dopamine*, and *serotonin*. These neurotransmitters, described below, will be mentioned several times in the course of the book.

A chemical rush

Norepinephrine is an excitatory neurotransmitter. It's a derivative of epinephrine—another word for adrenaline. Produced in deep regions of the brain, it travels along nerve cells to parts of the brain that cause your body to experience heightened sensations. Indeed, it's the rush of adrenaline that you associate with finding out you got into the college of your choice or when you win the lottery. Ironically, it's also the neurotransmitter involved when people get panic attacks or are confronted with a sudden threat to their life or limb: a physical rush of intense emotion, rapid heart rate, shallow breaths, skin flushing, butterflies in your stomach, and numbness in your fingers and toes.

If you think about it, that makes sense; the body rush you feel after winning a million dollars (not that many people actually know what that feeling is like) or when you are just seconds away from a head-on collision are quite similar. But, when you know that one adrenaline rush is associated with something good, you can relax about the weird feelings in your body. When the rush is associated with something bad, or when it comes out of the blue (as is the case of panic attacks), the uncomfortable bodily sensations send you a message to pay close attention.

Relationships work the same way; when you become infatuated with another person, not surprisingly, you experience a surge in norepinephrine. Poets have long written about the heady, floating, walking on air feeling that occurs when people fall in love. When Carole King croons, "I feel the earth move under my feet, I feel the sky tumbling down . . . whenever you're around," brain researchers would have no hesitation in concluding she is singing about the surge of norepinephrine that happens when infatuation takes hold.

The reward neurochemical

In the *raphe nuclei*, which are part of the brainstem, neurons produce a different brain chemical, called dopamine. This neurochemical travels from the brainstem, up through nerve cells, and spreads out to different parts of the cortex. Like norepinephrine, it is considered an excitatory neurochemical, as it turns on many kinds of brain activities. Dopamine mainly functions to regulate your brain's system level of alertness to pleasurable stimuli. Your dopamine levels lay low on a day-in-day-out basis. The daily drudgery of life doesn't do much to raise them up. But when something potentially delightful is about to happen (or is happening), dopamine chemicals pour out of your midbrain and saturate parts of your brain with a pins and needles kind of anticipatory excitement.

When your brain is exposed to dopamine, you have a strong physical sensation, not unlike what you feel with adrenaline. In fact, when the blood pressure of critically ill patients starts to fall to dangerously low levels, often doctors will order an injection of dopamine in order to shoot the blood pressure back up and revive the dying patient. That's exactly the kind of revitalizing power that dopamine can have to your body. As for its effects on the brain, consider that, when individuals lack dopamine (as in Parkinson disease), they slow down to a halt, and, when they have too much dopamine (as in schizophrenia), they may be agitated and have hallucinations.

How does all this relate to falling in love? When a new love object —a boyfriend or girlfriend—comes into your life, it pushes dopamine levels higher. The consequent heightened arousal and surge of positive emotions have a strong stimulating effect on the brain. You're ready for all good things to come your way.

♣ ONE NATION, UNDER PROZAC

When it comes to timing of my medical education, I couldn't have had it any better. When I graduated medical school in 1985, "tricyclic antidepressants" were the main medication treatment options available for patients with depression, and effective treatment improved people's moods, sleep, appetite, interest, and energy. These medications, still in use today, are believed to work through correcting the brain's chemical imbalances. But they affect the levels of many neurotransmitters, so, even when patients improved, doctors couldn't say exactly which brain chemicals were responsible for which reactions. Moreover, because these neurochemicals were affecting so many parts of the brain, people frequently complained bitterly of burdensome side effects. Some patients were unable to get to a high enough dose to help them because of adverse reactions.

Then along came a revolutionary new medication: Prozac. This brand name for fluoxetine hydrochloride was revolutionary, because studies suggested that it mainly acted on the levels of serotonin and no other neurochemical. Normally, serotonin production is so plentiful that brain cells recycle the leftovers by pulling any extra back into the neurons by a process called *reuptake*. Even though people with depression have lower than normal levels of serotonin, the vacuum cleaner–like process of reuptake continues unabated, thereby depleting the meager stores of serotonin. Prozac acted like a hand draped over the nozzle of a "reuptake" vacuum cleaner: by slowing down the recycle process of serotonin back into the neuron, Prozac caused more serotonin to be floating around for the nerve cells to use. Prozac fell into a new class of agents, *selective serotonin reuptake inhibitor*, or SSRI.

I remember the debates among psychiatrists. How would patients react to a medication that didn't affect whole handfuls of neurochemicals? Would only specific kinds of patients improve? Would patients only get partially better? Now, more than twenty-five years later, everyone knows the answer to the questions. Not only was Prozac just as effective as the tricyclics in the majority of individuals, but it was much better tolerated. We concluded that it was not necessary to flood the brain with all kind of neurochemicals; for many people, adjusting serotonin alone would do the trick.

With the new SSRI tool in hand, researchers went on to discover that psychiatric conditions such as obsessive compulsive disorder, panic disorder, social anxiety disorder, generalized anxiety disorder, posttraumatic stress disorder, bulimia, even premenstrual dysphoric disorder (a kind of premenstrual syndrome) could all be successfully treated with SSRIs. Because we believed that these medications increase levels of serotonin in the neurons, we concluded that depletion of serotonin caused a whole variety of psychiatric problems. Now, with Prozac (and other SSRI) prescriptions at the ready, psychiatrists were on the lookout for signs of low serotonin: restless sleep, eating problems, depression, listlessness, anxiety, worry, even obsessiveness were all treatable conditions.

❧ SERENE OR OBSESSED?

What does this have to do with love? We know what happens to the levels of energizing norepinephrine in the brain when people are in love—they go up. We know what happens to the levels of the alerting dopamine in the brain when people are in love—they go up. So, what do you think happens to the levels of the soothing and mood-elevating effects of serotonin when someone is in love?

They go down! When I first heard this medical finding I was dumbstruck. If being in love makes people happy, then wouldn't there be a huge rise in the very neurochemical synonymous with happiness—serotonin? But as I thought about it, I realized it made perfect sense. For, when you examine the behavior of someone who is bitten by the love bug, it is not the picture of contentment. People who are smitten have many of the characteristics of someone with low serotonin. They are obsessive (*It's been fifteen minutes since she last called me! My skin looks terrible; he won't want to go out with me again*). They are worried (*When will I see her again? Will he call me? What is he doing right now? What if she changes her mind?*). They lose sleep. They lose their appetite. And, often, unless they are actually in the company of the person with whom they are smitten, they are not even happy. Being in love is the opposite of calm and serene; it can be very disturbing.

When a new attractive person comes into your life, an affair can get sparked when the same neurochemical changes that fostered that "in love" feeling with your mate happen all over again. Here's a description from my Internet forum:

I am a smart, reliable, decent, wonderful mom, and a loving and caring housewife. I am turning 52, and I've been married for twenty-five years to the most wonderful guy. Not perfect, but I have no complaints. He is generous with gifts, even though not rich. Diamonds, travel abroad . . . just ask and he will try to give. He is a wonderful father, the kids love him, and I love him too.

Suddenly I met someone married and fell in love at first sight. I can't sleep, can't eat, just thinking about him, praying that he will feel the same.

The worst thing is I know I will lose everything. Nice beautiful house, wonderful kids, great loving husband, move to another country.

I have not one good reason to leave. And yet, given a chance (I asked deep in my heart), and if he felt the same as I do, I will turn my back to all I have and earned all these years and be with him, if only for a few years.

Why? Because for so many years I have not had these feeling of being in high school again, young silly woman in love. So what? I will be 60 in a few years. Why not enjoy my remaining few younger years?

Am I not normal?

Yes, she is normal. Even at 52 she can still feel like a teenager. That's what norepinephrine and dopamine can do. And as for the sleepless nights and pushing away the dinner plate, she has all the markings of being in a low serotonin state. Not only does this chemical cocktail affect emotions and energy, it affects judgment as well. It's hard, almost impossible, to make good judgments under the influence of such a strong neurochemical pull. Yet that's exactly what happens in every affair, and you need to know about it. (Granted, it happened during dating your spouse, also. But the process of falling in love, dating, getting engaged, and ultimately marrying is more thoroughly thought out, and it involves the feedback of many more people, than the process of having an affair does.)

❧ PHILOSOPHY, MEET PHYSIOLOGY

Many philosophers and spiritualists understand the experience of finding our one true love and clinging on to that person as a way of completing the self. On discussing love, Plato wrote how lovers start out as one being: "The form of each human being as a whole was round, with back and sides forming a circle, but it had four arms and an equal number of legs, and two faces exactly alike on a cylindrical neck; there was a single head for both faces, which faced in opposite directions, and four ears and two sets of pudenda."

He goes on to describe how this human form had enough power to overwhelm the gods, so Zeus cleaved the form in two. These two halves are thrown across the planet and spend their lives searching for the other.

Many people share the idea that incomplete "souls" wander the planet and only feel as one when they reunite by finding the one and only one soul meant for them. They can reach no other conclusion but this one: *This person must be my soul mate.* But looked at through the eyes of a neuroscientist, a low serotonin state of pining away generates an intense sense of incompleteness. This distressed state is immediately reversed when the object of affection (the person you are infatuated with) is in your presence. Arm in arm with that person, you feel an immediate rebalance of your neurochemicals: you sleep better, you worry less, your appetite picks up, and your tension goes down. You feel "complete." This neurochemical description, I admit, isn't nearly as romantic as Plato.

♣ QUENCHING THE FIRE OF DESIRE

I opened this chapter describing why people marry is not much different from understanding why people have affairs. Hormonal surges and fluctuating levels of neurochemicals don't just happen to people who have affairs; at one point or another, they happened to those very same people when they fell in love with their spouse. The only problem is that those feelings fade over time. I recall an episode of the 1970s TV series *All in the Family*, when the daughter, Gloria (played by Sally Struthers), is upset because she has problems generating the same level of passion for her husband, "Meathead" (Rob Reiner), as she did when they first met. She is shocked when her mother, Edith (Maureen Stapleton), tells her that it's normal to feel that way, because otherwise no one would ever get any work done. She's right, of course.

You can't sustain the kind of high dopamine, high norepinephrine, and low serotonin state of early love because other aspects of your life—from friendships, to work, to family commitments—would all stop. So you do what's normal: you settle down, propose, and marry, and over time you get into a routine with your mate, you start to feel comfortable and safe, your levels of excitatory neurochemicals drop, and levels of your relaxation transmitter, serotonin, pick up. And you're ready to move ahead in your life.

❧ INFATUATION VERSUS MATURE LOVE

During the attraction and the infatuation phases of love, our biology drives us through topsy-turvy neurochemical decision making. But, as *All in the Family*'s Edith Bunker points out, we don't remain slaves to these desires forever. At some point, usually anywhere from six months to two years, our brain chemicals return to normal balance. Does that mean that you fall out of love?

Yes and no. If you think "in love" is fireworks in the sky, butterflies in the stomach, and gazing into each other's eyes for the rest of your life, then, in most cases, being "in love" does end. That's one of the reasons why so many break-ups begin with the conversation, "I love you, but I'm not in love with you." When these words are uttered (and you may have spoken them to, or heard them from, your mate) the words "I love you" mean "we share a connection and history, and you are an important part of my life—like my family members and close friends." The implication, obviously, is that that kind of feeling simply isn't enough, and if you don't have the "in love" passion in the belly, then the marriage can't be sustained. It's a shame that so many people feel that the absence of infatuation proves a marriage is DOA. I, for one, don't believe that it is true.

What *is* true is that the kind of love that you feel in marriage shifts over time from the high-pitched excitement of "in love" to a more mature love. This is the kind of deep emotional connection we see in couples who have been married for many decades. He may not get an erection every time she walks into his study, and she may not thrill to see him across the dance floor at a charity ball. But they have a kind of closeness that is deeper than that of parents and siblings, coworkers, and friends.

Despite the dramatic change in the tenor of the love, brain chemicals still play a role. When couples stay together past the infatuation phase, the hormones oxytocin and testosterone (again) are in action. Testosterone levels actually fall in men who marry and again in men whose mate bears a child. It's thought that such a change in biology reduces a man's urge to hunt out new women, but, as you can imagine, it may cut down on the wild passion in his own den.

Oxytocin, a hormone produced in the brain's pituitary gland, was first discovered more than a century ago as the chemical responsible for the contraction of the uterus during childbirth. Later it was determined that oxytocin was the key hormone in the production of milk. Thus, oxytocin is responsible for producing and nurturing a child. As an added bonus, researchers have found that it also plays a large role in bonding to that child.

But oxytocin doesn't discriminate; it increases the sense of closeness and connection not only to a baby but to anyone connected to a high-oxytocin person. When experimental subjects are injected with oxytocin, they are willing to give out more money to strangers because they feel more trust. These heightened feelings of connection result in increased "bonding." Animal research with the prairie vole, a mouse-like rodent, shows that these animals have high oxytocin levels and strongly bond with their offspring and mate for life. Their cousins, the mountain voles, in contrast, have low oxytocin levels and can't recognize oxytocin in their brain; these animals form poor connections with their broods and ditch their partner moments after they mate. Unlike prairie voles, mountain voles are unable to form lifetime connections with any other voles.

Humans, all humans, have oxytocin. As a species, we are meant to form bonds with other members of our tribe. When two people shift from the high-arousal infatuation phase to the more mature love phase, the levels of oxytocin begin to rise. Generally, it is higher in women than in men, but men do have a mild surge during physical acts such as touching and a huge surge during orgasm. Thus, during these moments, men will feel an increased sense of bonding to their partner. (Unfortunately, this is also true for men when they experience orgasm with their paramours. They will have a high level of bonding and feel an increased sense of trust, duty, and commitment to the person they are not married to.) The low level of testosterone permits the oxytocin's effects to be felt even more strongly.

Gradually, a connection grows between two once wild-and-crazy lovebirds. You build a nest together and form a level of comfort and connection that is much deeper and, from my point of view, more meaningful, than the earlier phase of the relationship. This mature love must be recognized for what it is and not disregarded as evidence that you are no longer in love.

Does that mean that you are simply destined to become bored with each other, as you soak in your relatively mundane oxytocin baths? Absolutely not! As I discuss in chapter 11, you and your mate can do many things to bring titillation and energy to your marriage.

❧ ALL IN THE INSTINCTS?

Research reveals that during a lifetime the average man will have more sexual partners than the average woman. One of the reasons that males of any species are more likely to have sex with multiple partners is reproduction. Males have virtually no limit to how many sperm are available to them, and their bodies make no sacrifice in spreading their sperm around to healthy females. Not only that, but the more females a male fertilizes, the greater the chance that his DNA will live on. And in survival of the species, that's what it's all about.

From an evolutionary point of view, it doesn't make much sense for female mammals to have a lot of sex. A woman only produces an egg (ovulates) once a month; if she's not ovulating, she can't get pregnant. Moreover, when she gets pregnant, she can't get pregnant again until after she's given birth. Based on fertility, it would make sense for a woman to have sex maybe three days a month. Once a baby's on the way, there's no biological rationale for her to have sex for the next nine months. Yep, you heard me right: assuming she gets pregnant within three months of meeting a man, a woman's biology requires she has sex about nine days a year.

Unlike males, females have a big biological price to pay if they have sex. Whenever sex occurs, there's a chance that it could result in pregnancy, which can drain the female's nutritional status, blood supply, and calcium stores and leave her physically and mentally exhausted by years of raising her young.

At this point biological drive and social structure merge. Human babies, unlike most other mammals, are entirely helpless after birth. They can't even hold their heads up for several weeks. A baby giraffe, by contrast, can stand on its feet and join the herd within one hour of being born. Human females must hold their babies when nursing or nurse lying down, so their ability to seek food and defend themselves is severely inhibited. Many scientists believe that men and women couple and share the responsibility of raising the child because, unless they work together, the child will die. Thus, it appears that our social structure, like our sexual behavior, has roots in making sure our gene pool endures.

♣ PAIRING FOR LIFE

Does the drive to pair up and remain coupled during raising a child mean that humans are designed to be monogamous? Unfortunately, the animal kingdom doesn't have a whole lot of great examples of species that can boast a lifetime of bonding. It's inspiring to think of gibbon apes, otters, wolves, and coyotes as bonding for life. But only 3 to 5 percent of all mammals are monogamous. It had been thought that many bird species also bond for life, like eagles, vultures, and certain cranes. However, genetic studies are now showing that up to 30 percent of the eggs that the female bird sits on have DNA from birds other than their "sole" mate.

Perhaps the best animal kingdom example of a committed relationship is the anglerfish, which live in the deepest recesses of the ocean. If you've ever seen a photo of the anglerfish, you'll know that only another anglerfish could find it appealing. The male is much smaller than the female, and when he finds her through sense of smell, he bites into her side, where enzymes dissolve his skin and hers, fusing them together for life. Now that's commitment!

On an unconscious level your body knows these facts about the biology of sex. Your body is driven by these subliminal influences day in and day out. It is not just a myth that women pick strong-but-silent square-jawed He-Man-type guys as objects of sexual desire and then choose gentle, kind, and consistent men to marry and to help them raise children. When women are given hypothetical mating profiles, they prefer men who will be able to provide for the family and keep the family safe. Men, long disparaged for their propensity for seeing potential mates "only skin deep," tend to prefer women based on body shapes (the classic hourglass figure) that suggest reproductive ability. Even studies of 75-year-olds show that women seek sex for the purposes of emotional closeness, while men are interested in women whom they find good-looking.

Investigations into human biology take us one step further as we try to answer the question of whether there is an evolutionary advantage to the offspring for a man and woman to stay together for life. Some theorists support this idea. A woman's enjoyment of sex, even during times when she is not fertile, serves to keep her man as part of her life even when it doesn't involve baby making. This rewards and reinforces monogamy, because it gains the protection of the man over her and their offspring. The little ones will have an increased likelihood of surviving long enough to procreate, thereby carrying both parents' DNA into the next generation. And a faithful and loving mate, while having fewer offspring, can be more likely to raise those who are actually his.

There are arguments on the other side of the evolutionary question. Here experts explain why humans are not meant to stay together past the time when a baby takes its first steps (and the mother can again fend for herself). The father who produced this child can rely on the protective instincts of the woman to provide good survival odds for his child, while he goes out to seek other women to propagate his genes. The mother, once her baby is able to toddle, could find a younger and fitter man to better defend her children and have more healthy babies with (although she might run the risk of the new man mistreating children who do not carry his DNA). Perhaps monogamy made sense when humans rarely lived past age 40, but these days biology might push a man to seek out younger fertile woman once the mother of his other children becomes too old to have children. Recall that there is a survival advantage of reproducing as much as possible, and men can do that up until death. Actor Tony Randall fathered a child at 78, and Ramajit Raghav, an Indian field worker, holds the reputation of being the world's oldest father at the age of 96.

No one scientist can say for sure, but, as far as most anthropologists and biologists are concerned, there is no reason to think that humans were intended to couple for life. There may be ethical, religious, spiritual, moral, and practical reasons for monogamy, but, quite simply, science suggests that humans were not designed to be monogamous.

So can everyone finally relax and just say that infidelity is natural? Yes and no. I don't want anyone to put down this book with the mistaken impression that I believe biology excuses infidelity. Biological reasons cannot fully excuse anyone from any behavior that is within his or her control. It's not okay to steal food because of the biological sensation of appetite, nor is shooting a neighbor's barking dog permitted because of a biological need for sleep. Couples who have experienced infidelity often rack their brains to figure out how something so dreadful could have happened. Many want to blame biology. But that's not enough of a reason to explain such a complex and intentional behavior.

❧ WHY DO PEOPLE HAVE AFFAIRS?

One of the differences between humans and other species is the ability to think abstractly and understand ourselves. We have a psychology—an inner working of the mind that prompts us to do things like imagine the future, create rock and roll music, and read self-help books. Even very simple things may have different layers of psychological meaning, and each of these meanings can also go several layers deep.

Here are some of the psychological reasons why a person makes the decision to have an affair.

Reason 1: Having an affair makes someone feel attractive

I discussed the notion of "attractiveness" in chapter 1. The bottom line is that most people hope that others will see positive physical attributes in them and want to spend time with them. People place a lot of effort (and money) trying to be physically attractive. Financial experts estimate the value of the global beauty industry of skin care as $24 billion; make-up, $18 billion; hair-care products, $38 billion; and perfumes, $15 billion. And that's not including money spent on diets, gyms, and cosmetic surgery.

People want to be liked for things other than their skin and hair, of course. True beauty has to do with more than just physical features. Each of us questions our own attractiveness by asking, "Am I the kind of person other people like to be around?" "Am I funny?" or "Do people pay attention to the things I say?" We make efforts to be amusing, tell interesting stories, or act politely. We laugh at others' jokes and gawk at pictures of their children all in an effort to be the kind of person who others want to be around. When you walk into the room, are people happy you are there? If so, that helps you to feel attractive.

Despite all the talk these days about loving yourself (not that I disagree with the premise), the important thing to remember about attractiveness is that it is entirely dependent on perceptions of other people. That's included in the definition of the word—the capacity to draw others toward you. That is the only way you can measure your attractiveness: by observing the reactions of those around you.

People have an intrinsic desire to be attractive, and they will seek evidence of it in all people they meet. But the likeliest person to give them honest feedback about their attractiveness is their spouse. The reason two people marry is that each of them felt a tremendous attraction toward, and from, their spouse-to-be. That attraction was a turn-on. The newlyweds assumed that that attraction would continue, unabated, for the rest of their lives.

If I ran the world, I would insist everyone make daily efforts to assure his or her partner that she or he is attractive. I would also advise each member of a couple to look for ways in which your life partner may be showing attraction toward you, even if it's not obvious at first. But the reality is that, after a while, married partners begin to take each other for granted. Moreover, a phenomenon called *habituation* takes effect, in which so many of the things that delighted you become background noise. Your lack of awareness (of how pleasant, reliable, good natured, and sweet smelling your mate is) isn't a way of saying that you don't find him or her attractive, it's just a baseline, and you've come to expect it. When you no longer light up the room in response to your partner's good qualities, and when he or she no longer beams in response to yours, you each begin to feel less attractive.

Habituation happens in every marriage. Every young couple says it won't happen to them, but it does. Later in this book, I'll be talking about how to make consistent efforts to increase how attractive you make each other feel, but, for right now, I'd like to explain how habituation contributes to affairs.

Reason 2: Same ol' is same ol'

Familiarity

People in committed relationships take each other for granted because of habituation, bothersome habits, and exhaustion. When something is very familiar, it loses its specialness. That's why people want to buy new cars or new clothes, even when the items they have are perfectly fine. Even people who inherit wheelbarrows full of money grow tired of having everything they want. So it is with the special qualities of your mate: they lose your attention.

Annoying habits

Being together consistently over time also introduces you to more things you don't like about your mate. You may not have noticed when you were dating that she spends hours shopping on eBay or he always reloaded the dishwasher before running it. After you wed, though, these behaviors begin to capture your attention. Because you've accepted the positive as a matter of course (he shows up at the dinner table every night), you're more drawn to the negatives (he never puts his napkin in his lap). As marriage progresses, it becomes harder and harder to recognize the things about your mate that attracted you to him or her in the first place. But, if you were asked to write a list of reasons why he or she is unappealing, you'd complete it in no time.

Exhaustion

Sharing a household requires a lot of work, and it is often the kind of work that is least satisfying. Making the beds, washing the dishes, locking up the doors at night, and paying the bills are the kinds of tasks that happen every day. Emptying the cat litter box or complaining to the mechanic about his shoddy service drain the niceties out of daily life and rob couples of the positive energy that highlights each other's goodness. These things must get done, of course, but once you settle down with each other for the night, it's hard to feel attracted to the person who shared in your daily grind.

Reason 3: The allure of others

While the newness of your relationship may be fading, and with it the sense of animal magnetism you share for each other, the world is full of people who are new to you, whose bothersome ways you don't know about (and vice versa), with whom you share no drudgery. These people find you appealing and you, in turn, find them appealing right back. Your husband might groan when he hears your joke for the hundredth time, but your new coworker laughs with abandon. While your wife ignores your newly polished shoes, your boss comments on how spiffy you look. When another person reaches out to you and makes you feel like you're funny, cute, smart, or nice, that gets noticed. In fact, the experience is just the opposite of habituation—novel stimuli turn on brain chemicals (dopamine again!) and improve how well you pay attention.

Here the brain takes us through a natural chain reaction. When a person feels like he or she is pleasing to someone else, a natural attraction begins to emerge. It's the opposite of the Groucho Marx comment that he would never want to belong to any club that would have someone like him as a member; in fact, we are more attracted to the clubs that want us. Just the notion that someone thinks I'm extraordinary tells me that person must be special in some way; after all, he or she recognized *my* distinctive qualities.

Where marriage, by nature, results in a gradual waning of appeal, a new relationship is an alluring trap, one that will make you feel more attractive by the boatload.

Reason 4: Lack of morality

Why do some people amble over to the fruit stand, grab an apple, and run off? Why do some students pay a professional writer to finish a term paper for them? Why do some people forge checks from their grandmothers' accounts to buy sports cars? They do these things because they can. In most cases they know they should not, but no moral or ethical voice is telling them not to.

Most people have a sex drive, find other people desirable, and have some areas of dissatisfaction with their marriage. But most people don't justify breaking their marriage vows and sleeping with other people because of this. Some people, however, have affairs—as is the case with other liars, thieves, and cheaters—because they can. And that's all the reason they need.

Charmer or something worse?

The term *antisocial personality disorder* (ASPD, also known as socio-pathic disorder) is bandied about lately in the cable news shows, as pundits try to explain the soulless criminals who murder, rape, or kidnap people. The term is borrowed from psychiatry and is a diagnosis made when an individual has a pervasive pattern of behavior with symptoms that include the inability to conform to lawful behaviors, repeated lying or conning, aggressive and assaultive actions, reckless disregard for others' safety, and the inability to stick to one job or one relationship. These behaviors are compounded by the attitudes of the antisocial individual, who is indifferent to others' feelings, fails to show remorse, and lacks depth of feeling.

People with ASPD are often charismatic. They flatter, compliment, and nod in seeming sympathy with the person they are talking to. But unlike most people, who genuinely wish for mutual positive feelings to be shared by all, when sociopaths sweet-talk someone, they do it with only one thing in mind—getting their own needs met. Once that innocent victim has been used for the sociopath's purpose, he or she is ignored or betrayed by this once charming smooth talker. "Used and abused" would be the motto of anyone who has crossed paths with someone with antisocial personality disorder.

ASPD is considered a psychiatric disorder. People don't choose to have this problem any more than they choose to have schizophrenia or obsessive-compulsive disorder. People with ASPD have difficulties managing the demands of everyday living; they are prone to finding themselves in social difficulties, plagued with substance abuse, or even in prison. When sociopaths first get hired for work, they seem like the ideal employee. However, once the luster of their charm wears off, they can no longer hide their selfishness and irresponsibility from their bosses and wind up returning to the unemployment line.

Not everyone with ASPD fails to keep a job. Some people with the disorder, by virtue of their ability to screw over others with impunity, are quite successful in business and are at the top of the food chain in their corporate or professional lives. But a close look behind the scenes of their *Money* magazine cover stories reveals unhappy and unfulfilled personal lives riddled with multiple divorces, disgruntled ex-partners, and children who barely know their parent.

People with ASPD can't maintain relationships. They just can't understand about people's feelings. They have been told that they are supposed to empathize with others, but the concept is entirely foreign to them—they simply cannot imagine anything beyond their own immediate desires. They cannot feel guilt, pity, or even selfless love. They genuinely believe that their needs are paramount and that others exist on the planet for the sole purpose of granting their wishes.

Is every cheater a sociopath?

At some point during an affair, everyone lies and appears to have disregard of the feelings of the spouse—otherwise, he or she would never have started the affair in the first place. But most people have the ability to see, at least abstractly, that their actions have the potential of hurting other people's feelings. Many of the people with ASPD really just don't get it.

Let's take one example from a participant in my Internet community, William, 43 years old and married seventeen years.

I had an affair with a woman whose husband worked for me. She knew I was financially successful. Because of that, she went out of her way to make it convenient, only interested in pleasing me sexually, and telling me how great I was. She even took total responsibility to come on to me aggressively and set up every meeting, and everything we were to do, or what she would do for me. I just had to show up. The problem is that my wife is much more beautiful and loyal. She has a great body and is a perfect mother to our children. I sometimes would try to get mad at her, to feel less guilty about my infidelity, but she would try to accommodate me to get along. I *totally* love my wife; she just wanted me to show her more attention.

I was not sexually attracted to this other woman. I just wanted the worship she gave me. After we finally did have sex, I immediately ran out of her house and have not talked to her since.

You may have strong negative feelings about William's behavior. Like most affairs, it was self-serving and disrespectful to his marriage. He showed a shallowness of character in the way that he allowed himself to have sex with a woman he didn't care about. But was his behavior antisocial? William expressed guilt about his behavior, remorse for his bad decisions, and an appreciation of why his wife felt the way she did. These are all indications that, while William behaved indecently, he should not be labeled as a sociopath.

Contrast William's story with that of Ryan. I met 34-year-old Ryan when his 23-year-old bride, Jessica, came to me for a consultation. Ryan had let me know in no uncertain terms that he was not the problem in the relationship. Jessica had concerns about Ryan's seeing other women, but Ryan insisted that it was all in her mind.

In the course of couples' treatment, I usually meet with each partner individually. When I had my appointment with Ryan, he wove an intricate story about how he is fighting to save this, his *second* marriage. He described feeling misunderstood and a bit miffed that his wife didn't want him talking to other women. When I met with Jessica later that week, she told a different story. Ryan, she revealed, had lied to her about the fact he was already married when they first started dating. Further, before she had met Ryan, he had been arrested multiple times on various nonviolent charges. Jessica brought evidence to my office of Ryan's infidelity, including telephone records and discussions she had had with the women he was having an affair with—who confirmed Jessica's suspicions. And here was the kicker: Jessica revealed that this is Ryan's *fourth*—not his *second*—marriage!

When I later met with Ryan and Jessica together, I confronted Ryan about his egregious lie. "Why?" I asked Ryan, "Why did you say this was only your second marriage?" Ryan didn't seem embarrassed by the revelation of his deceit. He responded to my query nonchalantly: "I didn't want you to get a bad impression of me."

I got a very bad impression. Ryan lied. He lied to me, he lied to Jessica, and he was a liar long before he met either one of us. His ability to deceive others and blithely attempt to escape any responsibility for his actions suggested a lifetime of self-interest and lack of concern for the feelings of others. Ryan was concerned with one person, and one person only, even if it left other people hurt in his wake. In all probability, he was a sociopath.

A couple days after I confronted Ryan, I got a message from Jessica that the marriage had ended. I never saw either of them again.

Ryan's behavior shows how infidelity can happen when one partner has no moral compass and is concerned only about his or her own needs. We've already discussed how it is natural to find other people outside of marriage attractive. Lack of empathy for others gives the green light for any behaviors, even immoral or illegal acts, which advance the desires of the sociopath. And if that desire includes taking someone to bed outside of marriage, then infidelity is business as usual.

Not every marriage to a sociopath has to end in divorce, but it does require special awareness of the problem. In these cases, I recommend the spouse seek professional support to develop strategies for dealing with the effects of antisocial behavior on the family.

Reason 5: Addiction steers people off course

At the onset of treatment, I screen almost all of my patients for substance abuse. As part of that process, I ask a series of questions, many of which derive from recommendations of the Substance Abuse and Mental Health Services Administration.

Here are some of the questions from the intake survey (which uses the initials AOD as shorthand for "alcohol and other drugs"):

1 Have you tried to hide that you are using AOD?
2 Have your parents, family, partner, coworkers, classmates, or friends complained about your AOD use?
3 Has AOD use caused you to feel depressed, nervous, suspicious, uninterested in things, change your sexual desires, or cause other psychological problems?
4 Have you used AOD even though you knew it was keeping you

from meeting your responsibilities at home/school/work?

5   Have you needed more AOD to get the same high, or found that the same amount did not get you as high as it used to?

6   Have you had withdrawal problems from AOD?

7   Have you used any AOD to stop being sick or to avoid withdrawal problems?

8   Have you used AOD in larger amounts, more often, or for a longer time than you meant to?

9   Has AOD caused you to give up, reduce or have problems at important activities at home/socially/school/work?

10 Have you kept using AOD even after you knew it was causing or adding to medical, psychological, or emotional problems you were having?

The person who has an occasional drink, or periodically smokes a joint, tends to answer most of these questions with a "no." However, someone with a substance abuse disorder tends to say yes to almost all these questions. All sorts of people with all sorts of addictions begin to act in predictable ways that are typical of the disease of addiction. The behaviors go beyond having cravings for or withdrawal from a substance; they include hiding behaviors from others, lying about activities, investing time and money seeking a chemical high, and changing just about every aspect of one's life. Moreover, most of these individuals have wished to break away from their substances of abuse, but doing so has proved very difficult.

My work with addiction has led to a revelation that has affected what I do as a couples' therapist: Almost everything that happens to an addict happens to someone who commits infidelity.

What kind of addiction?

Infidelity is what I call a *flame addiction*. I am not talking about "sex addiction," because most affairs are about much more than sex. Affairs are about an internal chemistry stirred up by being with or thinking about the other person. What keeps people drawn toward each other is the intensity of the feeling. Once you get a taste of the burning desire—the flame—you're hooked.

When I think of flame addiction, I think about how candles attract moths. Moths move as near as possible to the candle's flame, circling in ever smaller loops, trying to get closer and closer. If you've had an affair, you know that the kind of attraction that you felt was no less intense, and no less misdirected, than a moth circling a candle. You may tell yourself that you ought to stop your misguided flight, but every time you move away from the flame you feel compelled to return.

A story of obsession

Rick contributed to my website and message board with the following story:

I met a woman whose child goes to the same school as my daughter. I noticed the woman right away and found her attractive even though she isn't my typical type.

During my daughter's kindergarten year, I'd see this woman, wild hair, purple streak, tattoos, ears completely pierced and a lip piercing. She'd sit at one end of the lobby and I'd stand at the other. I'd glance her way and never saw her look at me. I later found out her daughter and my daughter were best friends that year and into the oncoming year.

During the beginning of the first grade year, we talked a bit, began setting up play dates for the girls, and texting. My wife and I and her and her husband hung out as couples. I couldn't take my eyes off her body. She loved to work out and I am an avid bodybuilder. My wife at the time had let herself go somewhat, and it is absolutely no excuse for me to do what I did . . . but it's done and now I'm relaying it.

In March, it became known that she found me attractive and I let her know I felt the same. We agreed to meet and she said, "Let's have fun with this and see where it goes." Great, I thought, I've been married for fourteen years, and I've been curious about other women. Perfect! The next thing the other woman said was, "I promise you, I'm not crazy. I won't show up on your doorstep screaming and yelling." I should have run at this statement, but I plead ignorance.

So it started up, and everything was WOW! It felt right. We would go out on mini-dates during the day, and I felt like a kid again. We both acknowledged the newness factor and a few weeks in, she told me she was falling for me. That opened the floodgates, and I fell hard for her . . . or maybe it was infatuation.

We talked of leaving our spouses all the time, but she threw out another warning sign I ignored. She said that while she was in love with me, and that while we had a connection she had never had, she still loved her husband and wasn't ready to leave him . . . not yet. So I stupidly kept on, sneaking around to see her, and she sneaking around to see me.

Three months later, my wife found out, and I admitted to being in love with our "friend." My wife was devastated. I saw her pain but closed myself off to it. I felt distraught and mad that I lost my girlfriend, but also because I was going to lose my family: my daughter, who is my world.

Now, the other woman's husband doesn't know (my wife chose not to say anything), but during that time we still talked a bit. We talked about letting things cool down and being more careful and selective on how we meet. Then she texted me saying she couldn't do it anymore, her feelings of guilt were too great. After that, I was flooded with texts saying she couldn't stop seeing me, she loved me, and needed to see me once more. Then she would tell me that her husband was trying to do better, and in the next text she would tell me that she lied, things weren't really much improved. She said she had to try and make her marriage work, so that she knew she had given it her all.

The yoyo-ing went on for a bit, then I got hit with a no contact order. I felt horrible; I had no closure. I wanted to know if I was a game, if she truly loved me. Or was it just the excitement of the affair?

I contacted her and she told me she was happy to hear from me and then a few minutes later, bit my head off. This happened a couple of times and then all contact ceased. I was distraught and sought a therapist, both for my own needs and to save my marriage as my wife was/is willing.

The problem is, I can't stop thinking about her, knowing what I know, seeing what I've seen, even though I love my wife and want us to work, this other woman really made a profound impact on me and the way she ended things is probably more the issue than anything else.

Fast-forward to very recent. She tried to get me to meet her at the coffee shop, and I ignored it. Then, we both went out of town with our families not too long ago, and she initiated some contact, telling me it was beautiful where she was and she didn't want to come back. I responded with a one-word answer as my therapist recommended. I don't even respond at all sometimes. And several days later, I knew she was supposed to come home, so I sent her a text saying, "Back?" Her response was "Stalker, much?"

I went through the roof! Livid! After all she and I went through, shared with each other, a simple question to see that she made it home safe and I'm a stalker? !? So there it is. It's been weeks and no contact, none by her and none by me . . . yet I wish she would. Stupid, I know.

No, I will not rekindle the affair, even if she tries, I want my marriage to work, but I invested a large part of myself in the other woman and this all ended just three months ago, so it is fresh. I'm at a loss as to her behavior. If I run into her at the school, should I be worried that she will try to reestablish a connection, as my wife thinks she will?

Rick's experience is very much like the experience of others who have had affairs. He doesn't describe himself as someone obsessed with sex, nor does it seem like his connection to the other woman is based on sex alone. There is a rational part of Rick's mind that says, "This is wrong. I should stay away." In that vein, he ought to rejoice whenever this woman pulls away, since it should make separation easier. But the flame of attraction is very strong, and when he gets too far from it, he is pulled back.

After I read Rick's post, I had had a chance to correspond with him. Here's what I wrote:

Hi Rick,
Really, the question is not about her Jekyll/Hyde behaviors, it is (in my mind) about your behaviors. Your actions seem to be driven by obsession and

infatuation, piqued by the excitement of how exotic this woman is.

It feels great to feel loved, but it's not great to seek it in the wrong place. And for you, that means you have to break free of the obsessive impulses and recommit yourself to your family.

I didn't mention flame addiction to Rick, but I wanted to give him a clear message that he has lost control of his behavior and that it's his responsibility to get it back. Here's what he wrote to me:

I reread your response Doc, and one thing that stood out is that I am obsessed with her. I honestly fell for this woman and I fell fairly hard. I thought I saw a future for us and was literally going to walk away from my family to be with her.

I do love my wife, and I want us to work, and I know it will be difficult; it already is, especially for her. But there isn't a day that goes by that I don't think of the other woman. I miss her. I miss our friendship and the laughs we shared. It felt "right," as she used to say.

I'm an emotional wreck most of the time. Wanting to make my marriage work but torn because I wonder if I was supposed to be with the other one. It is the single worst thing I've ever done. The ramifications, both emotionally and physically, are more than I ever thought. I wish to God she hadn't ever said she found me attractive. I wish I were still content being in a rut in my marriage. I don't understand why I am obsessing over a woman who probably could care less about me and who wasn't mine to begin with.

About six weeks later, Rick wrote again:

I'm still troubled by not letting her go. I see her at times, she ignores my existence; there is no civility. I don't understand it and it still hurts. It's like being addicted to a drug and I'm tired of it. I don't know what to think, and, yes, I get the focus-on-my-marriage part but let's face it, as of now I'm having an unhealthy obsession with a woman who I built an emotional—and then physical—relationship with for about a year.

People who have affairs discover that the infatuation with another person can be as strong as the obsession for orgasm for a sex addict, or, for that matter, as strong as the drive for cocaine for a crack addict. How can we explain the emotional experience that leads a faithful companion to become obsessed, preoccupied, reckless, conniving, and depressed?

♣ THE NEUROTRANSMITTER-ADDICTION CONNECTION

We start by looking in the brain. I talked earlier about how dopamine and norepinephrine levels rise during the infatuation phase of a relationship. Recall that one of the main functions of dopamine is to regulate your brain's reward system. When you associate a pleasurable sensation (for instance a fragrant scent) with some outside experience (a rose), your dopamine system is forever primed to feel good when you are exposed to the event (whenever you see a rose, you get a wave of positive feelings).

Most of the time, the surge of dopamine in the brain is a good thing, especially when it's associated with positive desires. For instance, the brain scans of long-married couples who are deeply in love reveal that, when they see photos of their mate, dopamine centers light up. When the dopamine levels surge, these individuals have an overwhelming positive feeling, and they want to spend time with their partner. Dopamine gives the message to the brain to "Go get 'em! You'll be happy you did!" This idea isn't rational, and it's not well thought out. It's an irresistible gut feeling.

But the parts of the brain that are sensitive to dopamine can't tell whether the desires are healthy for the organism. Studies done with rats show that they will give up food and water for cocaine—and die as a consequence. It's thought that dopamine steered the rats in the wrong direction. Likewise, human heroin addicts have been found to have a surge in their dopamine when they see photos of matches, bent spoons, or bags of white powder. Although on a conscious level junkies know that using heroin can lead to deadly consequences, they nonetheless begin to feel a powerful urge to shoot up, even if they are in sobriety. You don't need to ingest a substance to feel a rush of dopamine. Research shows that it happens to gambling addicts when they are shown a deck of cards, lottery scratch tickets, or slot machines.

This flood of excitatory neurochemicals primes the brain for more and "better" things. When the happily married woman sees a photo of her husband, it produces a pleasing sensation, but also a sense of missing something (him). The really good feeling comes from being with him, and the high dopamine levels in the brain signal a drive to go find him. When the heroin addict has a rise in dopamine levels, he also feels excited and incomplete. His brain tells him that he'll only feel really right when he uses the drug.

Almost all addictions can be understood as irresistible cravings, and most experts agree that those cravings are mediated by dopamine. Flame addiction is no different. The person who wishes to end an affair might consciously tell himself or herself that things are over, once and for all. But any reminder of the other person—the voice, an e-mail, a picture, or even a memory—can generate a dopamine surge and start the avalanche of automatic feelings and the intense desire to be with that person.

And, as if a jolt of dopamine isn't enough to trigger an addiction, being infatuated with someone is complicated by another brain chemical we spoke about earlier, serotonin. Recall that the early phase of a relationship drives down the levels of this calming neurotransmitter and that low levels of serotonin are associated with obsessive-compulsive disorders and other impulse control problems. The combination of a dopamine drive and a tendency to become obsessed with something—well, that pretty much covers the behavior of someone having an affair.

From the Web: It's Not the Same as Meeting a Stranger

Many people probably experience thoughts of infidelity due to the lack of excitement in their marriages. Meeting someone else is risky, exciting, new, and fantastical. These factors rarely exist in a long-term, committed marriage. While I cannot act out any such fantasies of infidelity because of moral and religious reasons, I wish there were a way of experiencing such feelings with my husband, as I feel that I have fallen out of love with him. Reading romantic novels can sometimes satisfy short-term cravings of infidelity, but they perpetuate the desire in the long run. Only major catastrophes such as infidelity, separation, or other means of betrayal can accomplish the feelings of renewal with a spouse after getting back together, but it is still not the same as meeting a stranger to fall in love with.

—Rose, 27, married five years

♣ IS BIOLOGY DESTINY?

Here I want to talk directly to the person who has had the affair: Understanding the chemical basis for addiction helps you understand how a perfectly sane person can act insane sometimes. It explains how difficult it is to resist actions that will produce negative consequences. But it does not excuse the behavior. The crack addict with the most intense dopamine rush still has the choice to not use; the gambler with a powerful craving to buy a scratch ticket still has the responsibility not to buy it. Millions of alcoholics, gambling addicts, shopaholics, and drug addicts have stopped their addictive behaviors. Millions of people have had affairs. These people dealt with the same urges, desires, and brain-chemical surges that you have. They stopped. You can too.

To those who have been the victim of infidelity, I am not excusing your partner's affair, but I want you to understand that addictive behaviors are not turned off because someone simply wills them to stop. It is a process that happens over time, often in phases, but it can be done. I am not condoning your mate's behavior, but I am explaining how he or she may have hurt you, seemingly without thinking, because of this irrational drive. Moreover, there's a good chance that he or she has made a promise to stop having contact with the other person and has gone back on his or her word. That is often part of the process of beating flame addiction. Now you know.

♣ RICK REDUX

Keeping this in mind, let's revisit Rick's story above. Rick describes a fourteen-year marriage and more recently being "in a rut." He meets a woman totally unlike his wife, with purple hair and assorted piercings, and finds her attractive. He briefly asks himself, "What if?" but thinks little more about it. At this point, he is conscious of an increase in interest that could happen to just about anyone. And, like anyone else, if his brain had been investigated in an MRI scan, we might have found evidence of a brief boost in dopamine, since any form of novelty will trigger dopamine. But Rick never received any reward for his longings, no fire was ignited, and no flame addiction was created.

This changed in an instant when this woman said she found him interesting. After that, the presence of this woman stirred intense desire in him. He could not shake the thought of her. He would be distracted at home in anticipation of their next encounter. As he came closer and closer to a sexual liaison, he continued to look forward to meeting her.

When Rick could be with the object of his attraction, he felt enriched by the affair. The heroin addicts I treat will tell me when they first try the drug it makes them feel *better* than normal, then when they go back to reality, they don't feel right until they are high again. Rick's experience was so satisfying that, like the heroin addict, he could not feel the same sense of well-being unless he was with this woman again. With her, he felt the rush; without her, he began to yearn for her.

Rick's flame addiction took off fast. And, like other addicts, the cravings controlled his life. It went out of control, and reality came crashing in. Yes, he figures he should have seen the signs early on, but now he sees them loud and clear. But it's not easy to stop.

As addicts will tell you, recognizing that you have a problem is a big step toward fixing it, but that's not all it takes. You must take back control of your life in order to heal from an addiction. You can; that's what this book will help you do.

As you go through the rest of this book, remember that your affair is probably the product of many thoughts, needs, and behaviors—everything from obsessing about your affair mate to lying to your spouse—and it will take time to learn new ways of thinking and acting. People who have benefited from recovery programs often use strategies to cope as they work on their sobriety.

♣ CAN YOU BE CURED OF YOUR FLAME ADDICTION?

Some people are adamant about one point: that once someone has an addiction, they always have an addiction. In many cases, that is true. People whose lives have come to ruin because of alcohol, or who have lost several marriages and businesses because of gambling, may always have a strong desire to drink or go to a casino. They are never "cured" from their addiction. These individuals, particularly if they participate in a twelve-step program, view themselves as "in recovery," not "recovered." And for good reason: because of the consistent draw of their addiction, they can never attempt to engage in those acts again.

But some addictive behaviors can be cured, and the person can recover (not just be "in recovery"). One fascinating study on alcohol abuse shows that many individuals who had clear-cut addictive behaviors in their late teens and early twenties now live lives of normal social drinking. I know that when I was in my twenties I had a few friends who could not go a day without getting high, but once they got out of college and went to work they switched to casual marijuana use. Many of them quit altogether.

In this book I offer you hope that people can be cured from flame addiction. I am hopeful about your prognosis because a flame addiction is usually about one specific person who has produced addictive-like behaviors in you. That conduct doesn't have to generalize to every woman or man you see for the rest of your life. Having strayed once, you must always avoid situations where affairs might happen in the future, but it doesn't need to be a source of constant worry.

Whether you consider yourself on the way to recovery or on the way to a cure, several concepts in the field of substance abuse treatment can be useful to you. These concepts originated with Alcoholics Anonymous and have helped tens of millions of addicts around the world. I will adapt the concept to flame addiction, but, as you can tell, the words "alcohol addiction" or "drug addiction" would work just as well.

One day at a time

Sometimes when you give up your addiction, the idea of never being able to speak to, see, or hear from your flame seems too unbearable to endure. And the prospect of doing it forever is overwhelming. You may be inclined to tell yourself, "It's just impossible, so I might as well give up trying to stop seeing him/her" and reconnect with your flame. But being apart from your flame is much more tolerable if you just take it one day at a time. Saying to yourself, "For today, I won't make contact" is less likely to put you in a panic. Each day when you wake up, commit yourself to staying away from your flame for that day and continue to do this one day at a time.

Seek support

One of the hallmarks of the twelve-step program is its reliance on fellowship with people who have been through similar situations to yours and have found ways to recover. Likewise, group supports (such as Al-Anon) are used by people who are married to (or children of) addicts. The idea of finding help in the community is a good one. There are two kinds of support I would recommend for people who have a flame addiction: (1) friends and family and (2) professional counseling.

Friends and family

First, turn to close friends and family. You may be tempted to keep the entire episode of infidelity hidden from the people you care about. It does make sense not to share your experiences with everybody, since some people are likely to jump to conclusions, label those involved, or seek revenge. Also you may be concerned (for good reason) that, if you tell certain friends of your spouse, they will push your mate away from you and advise you or your spouse to run away just at the point when you want to reconcile. These friends have all the best intentions, but they may end up having a destructive effect on your marriage.

However, keeping mum builds up your sense of confusion and isolation and makes it harder to move forward. When you have no one to verbalize your problems to, you may feel that this is just between you and your spouse. But, let's face it, your spouse is not likely to be a passive listener when so much is at stake. Consider the following pointers when trying to decide who to involve, and how to involve them.

One or two close friends, or close family members, should be invited to serve as confidants to help think things through as you make sense of your situation. Try not to choose a friend who is the same sex as your partner, unless it is a family member or unless your partner acknowledges this person as a friend of the family. Your partner may object to your talking to anyone at all, but I do not believe this is a fair restriction. It's often the case that the partner who by nature prefers to keep things close to the chest is married to someone who loves to talk. Likewise, the partner who insists that you *must* talk to someone (and, worse, tells you who to talk to) may also be establishing unfair expectations for you. Deciding if you want to share, and who you want to share with, is your choice.

You should first ask your friends whether they can be supportive in the way you need them to be. Also let them know that, if the load becomes too great to bear, they need to tell you. It's no easy job being your friend when you are struggling so much, and people need to know that they can step back when they need to, and you won't be offended or hurt. Many people worry that their friends will feel taken advantage of. If you keep communications brief, and requests for support reasonable, you'll find that people like to give support. Think about what you would do for your friend if he or she were to need you. Keep in regular touch with your friends, by phone, text, or e-mail, at least two to three times a week, even if there is "nothing" to report. Regular communication makes it unnecessary to spend a lot of time filling them in when something notable happens. It will also make them feel like they are helping.

You should be careful, though, about sharing strong and broad-ranged feelings in writing, as your partner could misconstrue the words you send to your friend. For example, one patient of mine had e-mailed to a friend how upset he was when his wife asked him to sleep in the living room. When his wife found out that he had told his friend, an argument ensued because she didn't think that detail was anyone's business. You and your partner are stressed enough; reaching out for support from friends should be permitted as an area of privacy, and as important to you. But in doing so, you run the risk of alienating your partner, so you need to be sensitive to his or her feelings as well.

Professional help

Second, seek professional help. One of the areas of greatest controversy around my first book, *The Secrets of Happily Married Men*, was my chapter called "Beware of Therapy." I believe that many counselors who say they are capable of doing couples therapy may not have the proper skills to help you. I know this, because I had been one of those therapists myself. But the help you may need to deal with your flame addiction may not require a marriage therapist. Just about any therapist who is skilled in helping you understand your behavior (if you have committed infidelity) can help you understand your pain (if you have been the victim of the affair) or can be instrumental in processing the firestorm of your emotions.

Of course, finding a therapist trained in dealing with affairs might be best, but absolutely, at all costs, find a therapist who is pro-marriage. There are therapists who specialize in couples' work who have themselves been married (and divorced) three times. We can't know everyone's circumstances, but, all things being equal, I'd rather see a clinician who has stayed married and who may be able to share those skills with me. (This isn't to say that I believe that you, given your unique circumstances, should stay married. You'll have to make that choice for yourself. I'll talk more about that in chapter 10.) Too many therapists jump to the conclusion that you have a bad marriage, a bad spouse, or just bad luck. Trust me, unless you are the victim of domestic violence, you do not want to see a counselor who will label your partner as bad and talk you into leaving the union—even, as I've heard about, providing the telephone number of a divorce lawyer at the conclusion of the first visit.

A few questions, and perhaps a trial session, will help you figure out whether this therapist is good for you.

1. *Ask whether he or she takes a promarriage stance.* If the therapist doesn't know what you mean, or tells you he or she is neutral, that may be a red flag. I tell people I'm a big supporter of marriage. I tell them, "I didn't choose for you two to be married; you did. But now that you are, I can help you find a way to have the high quality marriage you are looking for."

2. *Ask the therapist if he or she is married, and if so, how many times.* Most of the marriage friendly therapists I know are willing to share some personal details of their lives, to help clients get a broad perspective on their situation. Many excellent marriage pros are in their second marriage, but if they have two divorces (or more) you may want to stay clear.

3. *See if the therapist tries to diagnose or label your partner* (for instance, with phrases such as "personality disorder," or "codependent"). This is a bad sign. You don't want a therapist who puts your spouse down

(even if you feel like doing some trash-talking yourself), because that will alienate you from your partner. Your friends, however, are free to call your partner every name in the book.

4. *Be aware that the early phases of infidelity need plenty of attention.* Just like treatment for any addiction, these elements need to be addressed in therapy immediately. If you meet with a therapist who shifts the focus away from the affair because he or she would like to spend many sessions reviewing your childhood experiences, you may be wasting time that would be better spent on talking about what's really on your mind: your marriage. Sometimes it's helpful for a therapist to learn about your own family of origin, but the result of session after session of such exploration may be more insight into your authentic self and no marriage left to go back to.

Serenity and patience

One of the most helpful aspects of the twelve-step recovery program is the overarching desire for the addict to seek inner peace as an alternative to the outer craving. The flame-addicted individual must be prepared to say, "Today I seek serenity, rather than seek ____." It means loving, craving, and working toward the tranquility that comes with taking control of your life. Almost every AA member can recite the serenity prayer by heart: "Grant me the Serenity to accept the things I cannot change, the Courage to change the things I can, and the Wisdom to know the difference." In the case of infidelity, you must muster the courage this prayer calls for, because things *can* change.

Research tells us that changing behavior is not easy. For long-term addictions, the average person must try to quit six times before he or she succeeds. People in recovery often slip, but, for many, slipping doesn't foretell a debacle or even a relapse. It may be a temporary misstep that can be self-corrected and that only briefly impedes progress. For instance, one of my patients, Brad, had had a brief affair with a married woman he met at a convention but successfully terminated his (first and only) affair after his wife, Ashley, discovered the truth.

They were both seeing me in therapy, and he had begun to refocus his attention on Ashley and their two teenage children. Six months after he patched things up with Ashley, he had an urge to send a text to this woman to "check in on her." As soon as he had done so, he regretted it. But Ashley had seen the text and filed for divorce the very next day.

Ashley didn't look at Brad's recovery as a process; instead, she interpreted his behavior as evidence of how untrustworthy he was, plain and simple. Brad and Ashley are now divorced, and after several brief attempts of trying to make things work with his affair partner, Brad has ended that relationship. Now, three years later Ashley admits that she acted rashly and wishes her family could be together again. But Brad has already remarried an old high-school classmate. Partners of flame-addicted individuals need to be sensitive to the inconvenient reality that there will sometimes be small slips, but that doesn't mean the situation is hopeless.

From the Web: Trying to Do the Right Thing

Well I've finally done the right thing, I've ended my two year affair with a married man, and part of me just wants to call him right now and say I made a mistake, that I love him. I know that's just the fear speaking, fear of being without him, but I guess I'm not really with him, never was.

It started after I met his wife, who then introduced me to her husband; his wife and I became friends of sorts within a group of other friends. First it was over the Internet flirty chat, which then became a kiss, stolen petting, to a full affair.

We both are married and have children. About a year ago, one of our messages was intercepted by his wife. Since then we have continued our relationship in secret, hiding, sneaking out when his wife is away, calling each other, all the usual crap.

I feel like a monster. I love my husband and child, he treats me like a princess, has given me everything a woman could possibly desire, is caring thoughtful, listens, I mean really listens. He has a wonderful job and provides for me. He has treated me better than I have ever known, and I feel like the worst person alive. I don't know why I have done this.

He doesn't know, no one does, and hiding it has been horrible. I feel like such a liar, the most ungrateful person known to man. Hiding it has killed me, has made me sick again. I was in remission for my bulimia but the guilt has eaten away at me so that now I feel worthless. I haven't slept a full night for over a year now, I'm a basket case.

But I sit here, crying over the man I've just only an hour ago ended my affair with and I miss already. What does that say about what kind of person I am?

I have never spoke about it, held it all in, and for those who think being the other woman is pleasant, it certainly isn't. It's a living hell. A hell I made myself I only have myself to blame.

It's over, no matter how much it hurts right now. I can't go back, only try to go forward, try to forgive myself. I need to start again, begin to try forget the other man, and claim my self-respect and dignity back.

Higher power

Another feature of twelve-step programs is the belief that one must call to a higher power to help oneself through addiction. Likewise, some people who have had affairs will find that, when they can reconnect to their own higher power (for most people this will be the God of their religious denomination), they find the courage and guidance to get themselves on track. Many people whose partners have cheated will also find comfort and purpose in their religious community.

Some clean and sober addicts will avoid AA because they don't see themselves as requiring any assistance from a higher power. They believe that they can use their own mind and nonspiritual resources to heal their addiction. These people may seek help from groups (such as SMART Recovery), therapists, medications, books, meditation, or physical activity to get them through the worst of their addiction. Cigarette smokers make up such a group; while smoking is extremely difficult to quit, most ex-smokers have not needed to turn to a higher power to master their addiction.

Here is my advice: if you can find strength in turning toward religion, then make the effort to seek out your local spiritual leader. Religious attunement can have tremendous healing powers. If, however, you find that approach unhelpful, you still have many resources to aid your recovery at your fingertips. There are many paths to overcoming flame addiction; the important thing is not to lose sight of your goal.

From the Web: Rediscovering Each Other

We have rediscovered our needs for everyday intimacy—not just in the bedroom but also in the ordinary little happenings of seeking out what the other needs to feel good about ourselves. It took long, hard years of working things out together during the tough times, but always clinging to the fact that we knew in our hearts that we loved each other deeply and wanted to be together forever. Couples today don't give themselves time to grow old together. We thank God every day for the grace he has given us to hang in there and now we thank him that he has graced our lives with this time to continue to deepen our love for each other.

—Ellie, 65, married forty-five years

❧ THE COMPLEX HUMAN MIND (AND BODY)

Decades of scientific research into dating, attraction, marriage, and infidelity have yet to uncover one overriding reason why people cheat. In addition to the reasons described above, studies have pointed to the social expectations of the community, genetics (those who have an identical sibling who strays have twice the average rate of infidelity), or having an unfaithful parent. It's not likely that future studies will uncover one particular reason why some people cheat and some don't. But ultimately, the risks of infidelity go up when factors combine in a way that opens the doors to an affair. That's what we'll look at in the next chapter.

5

Giving the NOD to an Affair

IN THE LAST CHAPTER, I offered different explanations for why people look for and find love inside and outside of marriage. Everyone has hormones, everyone has biological drives, and everyone feels attractions to other people. But not everyone cheats. As many of the stories included in this book emphasize, cheating happens when a perfect storm of several factors come together. This chapter explores these factors.

🍀 A TIGER'S TALE

Let's start by looking at a real-life example of infidelity. Consider Tiger Woods, one of the greatest golfers, and possibly one of the most notorious philanderers, of our age. I've never met Tiger, so I am basing my profile on television and print information.

Tiger married Elin Nordgren, a Swedish model, in 2004, three years after he met her at a golf tournament. They moved to an estate just outside Orlando and had two children, one in 2008 and the other a year later. Just three months after the birth of their second child, Tiger ran his car into a mailbox just outside his driveway. Because of a *National Enquirer* article about an affair between Tiger and a nightclub manager named Rachel Uchitel, the press suspected that the accident was related to a fight between Mr. and Mrs. Woods. But nobody was talking.

By the end of the week, the silence was broken. Not by Tiger, or Elin, or even Rachel, but by a cocktail waitress named Jaimee Grubbs who claimed that she had been sleeping with Tiger for more than two years. By way of proof, she released the now-famous voicemail recording of a man she claimed was the star golfer saying: "Hey it's Tiger, I need you to do me a huge favor. Can you please take my name off your phone? My wife went through my phone. . . You got to do this for me. Huge. Quickly. Bye."

In the month that followed, eighty-nine different women came forward to proclaim that they had had sex with Tiger while he was married. By then Tiger admitted to having had an affair. According to one newspaper (the *National Enquirer* again), Elin finally decided to file for divorce in June 2010, when Tiger revealed he had a one-night stand with his 21-year-old neighbor, whom he had known since she was 14.

In a one-year retrospective on Tiger's infidelity published in a Tampa newspaper, thirteen women were confirmed as objects of Tiger's philandering, including porn stars, nightclub owners, social-ites, and a waitress at a Perkins restaurant in Orlando.

It's absolutely true that few people are as rich and famous as Tiger Woods. So his affairs may be much, much different from the affair (or affairs) that affected you. Tiger's story illustrates a fundamental certainty, however: for any affair to take place there must be three elements in play: a *need*, an *opportunity*, and *disinhibition* of impulses. The first three letters of these words, combined, give the NOD to an affair. In this chapter, I'll talk about how these three elements form the building blocks of cheating.

♣ NEEDS

As soon as most people cross the line into adultery, they begin to try to understand why they are attracted to someone outside the marriage and what needs their own spouse is unable to meet. After discovering an affair, the hurt partner often asks, "Did the affair happen because of something I did wrong, because of some way I was just not good enough?" I find that people who have affairs, and the people married to them, spend extraordinary amounts of energy trying to figure out what *exactly* the partner needed that wasn't being provided. Too much energy, in my opinion. The reality is that all of us have needs that our partner will not be able to meet.

Unmet needs unveiled

I have one patient, Eric, who gets great erotic pleasure when a woman intertwines toes with him. Not the most bizarre erotic fantasy, but it works for him. Eric's wife, in contrast, says she has very sensitive feet. Touching any living thing with her toes gives her the creeps, and she will not, under any circumstances, touch toes with Eric. Is Eric's need to have toes linked an adequate reason for finding another lover?

Eric is a reasonable guy, and he wouldn't risk wrecking his marriage over this issue. "It's not life or death for me," he says. But what about the following perceived needs, which *have* driven people to have an affair?

"I need more sex."
"I need different kinds of sex from what I'm getting."
"I need more attention."
"I need to feel needed."
"I need to feel special."
"I need to feel powerful."
"I need to be swept away."
"I need to prove that I can still wow a woman."
"I need to prove that I am still seductive."

"I need excitement in my life."

"I need to punish my partner for something he or she did."

"I need to individuate myself from my partner."

"I need to get my partner more interested in me by stirring up jealousy."

Getting needs met

Which of the needs listed above is sufficient to explain adultery? Which might someone like Tiger Woods have experienced? We can't know for sure, maybe even Tiger doesn't know, but I'd place a strong bet that he may have felt the need for sex, the need to feel special, to need to feel powerful, and the need to feel excitement. But you don't have to spend years studying human behavior to come to that conclusion, because many people who have affairs have the exact same needs. And if you really think about it, many people who *don't* have affairs have those same needs as well.

From the Web: Consolation Prize?

My wife hooked up with her first love from high school, who wrote to her through classmates.com. A long-distance affair that lasted about ten months. She got pregnant and called me while I was on business in Europe telling me she wanted a divorce. We have two girls in elementary school. I was shocked. She filed papers.

Somehow, we managed to stay together and cancel the divorce. Good thing she lost the baby, and he dumped her. Am I a consolation prize?

She tells me I don't communicate. I'm not positive and upbeat all the time. I don't hear her. I'm not emotional enough. Sounds like every marriage.

I've changed in ways she wanted me to. Things seem much better in the last couple months, but something inside makes me want to go out and just screw the crap out of some kinky babe. I would do it discreetly. I don't want a relationship. Just a torrid short-term affair. Will that mess me up? I don't know. But I still feel like I need it. Revenge? Consolation? Meeting the sexual need that is important to me and not to her?

—Josh, 39, married nine years

The factors related to needs that lead to extramarital relationships fall into three categories: a need for nurturing, a need for excitement, and confusion over needs.

Category 1: Need for nurturing

In my book *The Secrets of Happily Married Women* I write that men need nurturing. Many women e-mailed or came up to me after lectures to ask, "What about women? Don't we need nurturing too?" The answer, of course, is yes. While research suggests that a woman's style of nurturing might look different from that of a man, I have no doubt that both sexes need to feel cared for by those they are close to.

When I think of nurturing, I think of how a wife might provide comfort and assistance to her husband after a heart attack. In this case, nurturing means being cared for. I'm sure you can think of events in your lives when you were under the weather, either physically or emotionally, and someone you loved stepped in and reduced your suffering. They nurtured you back to health.

Nurturing can also relate to supporting someone's hobbies, goals, or aspirations. It's the Miracle-Gro that one person sprays on the dreams of another. I recall how one husband supported his partner's dream of opening up a boutique by helping her shop for fixtures and by painting the store walls. His partner felt taken care of by these acts.

Unlike attractiveness, which exists in casual and romantic relationships, nurturing either comes from professional caregivers (like psychotherapists, nurses, or physical therapists) or from intimate relationships (like family members or close friends). Most people in committed relationships seek the majority of nurturing from their mate. In fact, not only do partners desire that from their mate, they *expect* it.

As relationships settle into routines, husbands and wives become distracted and less attentive to their spouses. The mutual nurturing that came automatically now comes less spontaneously or not at all. Often the introduction of a child into the marriage will shift the balance, so that a new mother will pay close attention to all that her baby requires and be less focused on her husband's needs. Husbands, particularly those going to work while the mother stays home (if even for a few months), tend to increase their work hours and experience a rise in anxiety about income; they may have less tenderness to give their wives.

When nurture-seeking is the psychological motivation behind an affair, the partner who strays finds a new partner who makes him or her feel supported and comforted. That new partner expresses deep compassion for, and understanding of, unmet needs. This nurturing boosts the spirit and elevates the sense of self-worth of the person. He or she feels cared about and cared for. Hence, a sentiment that is supposed to be only shared with an intimate is now shared with an outsider.

Category 2: Need for excitement

I met with a friend, Nicole, over a cup of coffee when she told me about her difficulties with her relationship. She is a successful lawyer and her husband is an investment banker. They are each in their mid-thirties and have two young children. Over the years of their marriage, they had a rock-steady life: predictable, reliable, and turmoil-free. Nicole expressed a desire to do different and exciting things. She wanted to go to an adult-only Caribbean resort that catered to free-thinking liberal-minded clients. This was a loosely disguised invitation to "swing," or have sexual relationships with other married couples. Nicole's husband turned her down, and she was frustrated by his lack of consideration of her needs. "I feel like a caged animal," she confided to me. "Was this how I was destined to live my life, with the same boring hotels on the same boring beaches? I want something to pique my interest. I want our marriage to be an adventure, a pleasure journey, and he just doesn't want to come on board."

Nicole went through something that every couple experiences: after a while marriage tends to be less exciting. There are fewer mysteries, fewer surprises, and sometimes it seems like you could complete each other's sentences. In contrast, think about dating. Remember when you met, exchanged phone numbers or Facebook pages and wondered whether you would ever hear from that cutie again? Let me remind you: you were sitting on pins and needles. And then the next date you spent hours either putting on makeup or clearing all the junk out of your car or both. The newness of things ratchets up the level of interest. Every similarity interests you, "You mean you like Kings of Leon?" and every difference fascinates you, "You really don't believe in recycling?!"

Using brain scan images, scientists have peered deep into the brains of humans to try to figure how we make the decisions that we do, and without exception their studies have shown that new and interesting things stimulate the brain chemical dopamine, which causes a sense of euphoria. As we discussed in chapter 4, the infatuation phase of love causes a surge of brain chemicals that is indistinguishable from the changes that happen when a person smokes crack cocaine. When a man or woman who has no intention of starting an affair meets a man or woman who would like nothing more than to rip that person's clothes off, it literally causes a rush. Because marriages don't, as a rule, keep producing that cocaine-high of infatuation, meeting someone new may lead a person to do things that are out of character. That amazing buzz of being with a person outside of marriage has all the gratification, and danger, of a drug.

In Nicole's case, she wanted to control the level of excitement and invited her husband to partake in it with her. In chapter 11, we'll look at how couples can increase the feelings of excitement in their marriage. Nicole's idea for solving the problem didn't sit well with her husband (and would not have sat well with me had I been in his shoes). Rather than have an affair, Nicole chose to divorce her husband and seek out new partners who shared her ideas for a passionate adventure.

From the Web: Feeling the Butterflies Again

I am a 23-year-old woman, educated, beautiful and single. I attract many men, both single and married, although I find that married men are usually a lot more fun, since they would do almost anything for me . . . and the sex is usually great, since they are not getting any at home, or are getting some, but not fulfilling sex. Believe me, married men have the wildest fantasies. One married man I know calls it "repressed bedroom fantasies."

Mostly, I meet married men on the Internet. I cannot begin to tell you how many married men are on the Internet, especially when they are at their offices or at home late at night when their wives are asleep. I'd say a lot of these men love their wives but are looking for excitement. One man told me that he wanted to "feel the butterflies" again. A lot of married men just want sex with a younger woman, and they are quite frank about it.

Category 3: Confusion over needs

Life has lots of options. That's usually a good thing. But new research into the nature of human decision making has revealed a surprising finding: the more options you have in life, the unhappier you are. In one study, a group of people were told that they could choose one of two pieces of art as a gift, while another group was given a dozen artworks from which they only could choose one. Each person would go home with his or her selection. Later that day, when asked how happy they were with their choice, people with only two choices were found to be happier than those who had many more to choose from. How could that be? Simply put, the subjects who had many choices ended up leaving the experiment with the nagging feeling that they missed something. Research shows that the same thing is true of restaurant menus, clothing styles, and paint colors—too many choices leave people feeling regret over what they didn't choose.

It would be hard to conduct an experiment about the effect of choices on relationships. What might come closest are the popular reality TV shows *The Bachelor* and *The Bachelorette*. In these shows, an incredibly attractive man (or woman) is matched up with about twenty-five incredibly attractive women (or men). In the shows, the mission is to use multiple group and individual dates, make-out sessions, visits to meet the parents, and walks on the beach to winnow down the choices and find one true match. This situation might seem the answer to everyone's dream—more choices in one room than you are likely to get over a lifetime. Surely, with so many to choose from, the odds are that you'll find the love of your life, no? No. Fewer than 20 percent of couples on this TV series have stayed together for more than a few weeks after the end of the show.

Many people may see their lives as a reality TV game show, a real-life "Let's Make a Deal" and live under the constant impression that there's something better behind another door. The compulsion to seek something better at each opportunity raises the important question: What do you need?

From the Web: Childhood Issues

I have been unfaithful several times in my present marriage. I was caught. I know it has caused irreparable harm to our relationship. What is most perplexing is that my wife is wonderful—fun, beautiful, caring, sexy, a great mother, funny, a friend . . . everything.

My issues are from my childhood. My mother committing suicide when I was ten. I have always been afraid to commit. I have always been unfaithful. I have always pushed away those who love me . . . before they left me. Abandonment is a major issue in my life.

My wife and I are still together two years after the discovery. She is a saint. I am not. We have two wonderful children. We are working very, very hard at staying together and bringing back some or most of what we thought we had.

—Rufus, 47, twelve years into his third marriage

A hierarchy of needs

One of the primary tasks put before research psychologists is to figure out basic human needs. Perhaps the most famous work on the subject is that of Abraham Maslow, who constructed a theoretical pyramid made of five levels of human needs. Each higher level on the pyramid represents a need that is more complex and more difficult to obtain. The foundation of Maslow's pyramid was basic stuff of life, like breathing, eating, and safety from predators. In the middle of the pyramid Maslow places social needs, such as companionship and family. The tier second from the top represents self-esteem (characterized by self-confidence and respect from others) and the tip of the pyramid is the oh-so-difficult-to-achieve "self-actualization," an amalgam of morality, creativity, serenity, and generosity of spirit.

According to Maslow and many generations of psychologists who have followed, human needs are complex. In many societies where it is a struggle to find shelter or food, there's not much thought about self-esteem or creativity. As societies get more advanced, many of the basics are taken for granted, and people begin to seek more out of life than just finding food. For most humans during most of history, getting to the middle tier was about as good as it gets. Having a life partner, bearing and raising children, and being surrounded by family were sources of tremendous satisfaction. Now, however, a relationship that churns out kids and sets up a household just isn't gratifying enough. People seek fulfillment at the "self-esteem" and "self-actualization" levels, and they look carefully at their mate and ask themselves whether the wagon they hitched their future to will help them to get there.

There's a problem with expecting other people to bring you to higher levels on the Maslow pyramid: you can't rely on another person to "self-" anything. I dealt with that very issue when I treated a couple who sought therapy for their marriage problems. John was crazy about his wife and two middle-school-aged kids. He was a dynamic and well-spoken successful consultant who helped rescue businesses that were going down the tubes. He coached a high school debate team and ran his own "future business leaders" seminars after school. He earned more than twice what his wife Cheryl earned, and they could comfortably afford a nice home in the tony part of town.

In the year before seeing me, Cheryl had been asked to accept a special position working on new projects as a public school administrator. As Cheryl was exposed to more opportunities and more people, she began to gain respect and appreciation from her peers all over the region. She started to feel that John was not able to measure up to the amazing people she was meeting at conferences. These people made her feel great. She couldn't connect with John, and that made her feel unfulfilled in her marriage.

As I met with John and Cheryl over several sessions, I was reminded of Maslow's concepts, and how John looked toward the marriage as meeting his basic needs for family. He didn't need or expect Cheryl to "complete" him. John felt good about himself through his work outside of his relationship with Cheryl. While Cheryl got much satisfaction in her new role at work, she felt she could not advance to the next pyramid level of self-esteem if John were not able to help her get there. She saw John as holding her back from her goals of attaining the highest plane of self-actualization.

John was willing to try. After all, he was successful at his job and his coaching, and surely these roles require the ability to communicate. But John's well-honed verbal skills in the workplace had no effect on Cheryl, who continued to complain of not being understood by John, not being able to have a deep and meaningful conversation with him.

Cheryl's frustrations led her to the conclusion that someone else would be able to help her achieve these goals, and she began a long-distance affair with a man she saw when she went to conferences. Temporarily Cheryl was thrilled with the outcome, as she felt energized by the attentions of this interesting and interested man. But ultimately her goal of self-actualization backfired, as the relationship complicated her marriage and jeopardized the stability of the family. Rather than feel more elevated, Cheryl ended up feeling despondent over the direction her life was taking. She realized that, for her, an affair would never serve to fill her needs. She recognized that if she were to become happy in her marriage, she needed to change her expectations of what John could—and couldn't—do for her. She understood that the man she had slept with could not raise her self esteem. Her breakthrough in therapy came when she saw that what she needed most of all, she had to do for herself.

Ultimately "needs" alone don't suffice to explain affairs. In situations where unmet needs are at a boiling point, affairs can't happen until there is a way to have those needs met. That's where opportunity comes in.

From the Web: "Learning to like me first"

I have been married twice and have been unfaithful in both marriages. I had a need to be loved because I thought I wasn't. I don't understand the need but I am learning to like me first, and not depend on someone else to fill that need.

—Sharon, 43, in her second marriage

❧ OPPORTUNITY

Have you ever noticed that when Hollywood stars announce their newest love interest (whether they are already married or not), it's usually with the costar of their newest movie? When a recording artist announces a new whirlwind romance, it's very frequently with one of the backup dancers from his or her latest music video. Or when a male politician cheats on his wife, it tends to be with a member of his staff or press corps. That's because affairs are like real estate: The three most important elements are location, location, location. If no one's around to cheat with, cheating simply will not take place.

From the Web: "A secret life"

I met this married man six years ago on my job. As time went on, I noticed he was coming back into the salon on a regular basis requesting me for a haircut. I started noticing the eye-to-eye contact and found myself becoming really attracted to him. The sparks started to fly. The feeling was mutual. After about a year of flirting, getting to know each other, we started having an affair. Sometimes we meet for lunch to share stories and laugh, and other times it's very intimate. Our personalities are a lot alike, and he says he loves to be around me, says I always put a grin on his face. He's told me that if I ever stopped seeing him it would break his heart. Guess this is a secret life that two people can lead.

—Teresa, 37, never married

Finding an affair partner

People who have unmet emotional needs don't usually say to themselves: "I'd better start hanging out in some new supermarket (or bowling alley or soccer field) so I can find someone new to quench my unmet needs." No, most people who are prone to having affairs do what they normally do—they go to work, go to the gym, go to church, or go to the parent-teacher association meeting—and they typically don't go with the intent of having an affair. But if the opportunity presents itself, they might just get involved in something they never planned on.

We can't get into Tiger Woods's mind and figure out what his needs were, but we can get a look at his GPS and see where's he's been. And what we find is that all, or nearly all, of the women Tiger allegedly ended up having affairs with were women he met in the course of his day-to-day activities. They reportedly were from the neighborhood (in one case from across the street), the restaurants he ate in, the parties he went to, or the people he met through friends.

In your life, too, the odds are that an affair happened because two people were in the "right" place at the "right" time. Let's take a look at the locations that most frequently lead to an affair:

Bars or nightclubs
The workplace or classroom
Business meetings and conventions
The neighborhood
Class reunions
Facebook or other social network sites
Sporting events or concerts
The gym

The world's a big place, and there are many, many more situations, opportunities, and locations where people can meet; the important thing to realize is that affairs often happen because there is a chance for them to take place. I'm reminded of a song Cat Stevens recorded called "Another Saturday Night": "If I could meet 'em I could get 'em, as yet I haven't met 'em, that's why I'm in the state I'm in." Plain and simple, affairs happen because you "met 'em."

Proximity, need, and infidelity

Here's an example from an article about women and infidelity in *Newsweek* magazine. In this piece, Mike Torchia writes that in his thirty years as a Hollywood-based personal trainer, he has probably had affairs with more than forty married women. "Most of them were in their 30s, married eight to ten years, with kids, and their husbands weren't paying attention to them."

According to Mike, who's a trainer, not a shrink, women wanted more attention than they were getting. Recall that "more attention" was one of the needs listed earlier in this chapter. So if, indeed, the women who train with Mike feel this need, how do they end up with Mike? Because he's there. Mike tells *Newsweek*, "It's natural to want to have sex with your trainer. Remember that training is very hands-on. I'm touching them, motivating them, encouraging them, listening to them, relieving their stress, and channeling their energy in a more positive way. Just as their husbands used to do at the beginning of their marriage."

Geographic infidelity

Certain occupations are loaded with the opportunity to cheat. When individuals are away from their families for an extended time among others in a similar situation (such as the foreign service, military bases, or even prisons), a culture of on-site infidelity can occur when everybody involved understands that whatever emotional or sexual connection they have with another will be nullified once they return to their real homes and real lives. These relationships can be transient (as when one group of recruits stays in a barracks for a few weeks before shipping out) or more longstanding (as when two people are stationed overseas together over long periods). In many cases, the spouses of people involved in these affairs are never aware of their partner's "other life."

Electrical connections

Opportunity knocks not only on real doors but on virtual ones as well. One of the biggest changes in infidelity over the past two decades has been the availability of the Internet. I mentioned chance meetings in parent-teacher association meetings. But, at any one time, for every person sitting in a school cafeteria for a PTA meeting, there are hundreds of thousands sitting in front of a computer monitor, and these people are meeting each other at unprecedented rates.

Even before social networking sites, the Internet provided people opportunities to interact and communicate with each other. Simply joining sites for gaming, discussions, or information often connects you with people who make themselves intimately available. In these cases getting to know someone is accidental. But chance intimacy can be exciting, and it gives the illusion that fate has somehow played a role in the connection. That feeling of excitement can lead to decisions to get to know each other better, which step by imperceptible step can lead to infidelity.

A blast from the past

E-meetings don't have to be random to create the exhilaration of connection. Many of my patients have described how they joined social networking sites searching for old friends or how old friends have sought them out. Facebook is popular because it makes it easy to find a person by name and face and usually has links to your high school, college, or work—all the past places where you met that person in real life. In almost no time you can begin to rebuild your connection with your long-lost friend and tell yourself you can begin where you left off.

Bernie was one such person. I had been treating Bernie for his depression for more than five years. In that time, I had come to know him as a gentle and thoughtful man. He had recently celebrated his thirtieth anniversary and had successfully managed several stores in a chain of pharmacies. He had a stable marriage, and, while he stated he no longer felt any sexual attraction to his wife, he still loved her and had no thoughts about leaving her, "We have too much history."

One day Bernie went online to see if he could find his old high school girlfriend. Within a half hour he tracked down Ellen and sent her an e-mail. She e-mailed Bernie back the next day. She, too, was married with children. Their correspondence sparked a fire in Bernie. He e-mailed her more frequently, and his interest heightened. "What if?" he began to wonder. When Bernie discussed the interaction during our session, he heard from me the same advice I have mapped out in this book: a secretive relationship is dangerous and disrespectful to his wife, even though she doesn't know about it. If it ends up in an affair, it will be even more destructive.

During the first part of our session, Bernie tried to minimize and rationalize his behavior, saying, essentially, "Nothing's happened so far, so I'm not doing anything wrong." But, when asked if he might take things to the next step if Ellen proposed a liaison, he reflected on his sexless marriage and asked me, "What would be the harm?" In the style of psychiatrists everywhere, I raised my eyebrows and looked back at him and let him try to answer for himself.

When Bernie returned for a visit the following month he talked about his work, his children, and his parents. But he didn't mention Ellen. As the session wound to a close, I brought up his old high school sweetheart, asking whether they had been in touch much since our last session. "Ellen?" he asked. "No, I decided to end our e-mail communication. I realized that by keeping a fantasy relationship alive, I would hurt my wife and sacrifice my marriage." Bernie saw a potential opportunity to begin an illicit relationship but was able to control his yearning for an old flame and maturely put the potential affair behind him.

❧ DISINHIBITION

Clem of the Manor

When my family moved to a farm in the 1970s, we acquired our first dog, named "Clem of the Manor." Clem was a stately Labrador retriever—big, strong, and always hungry. Clem came from champion stock, but to us he was always just a member of the family. He was an outdoor dog, and he liked to wander onto neighboring farms when unattended. Needless to say, the other farmers didn't like that much.

So when we went out, we had to make sure he was penned properly. Clem did not like to be locked up. When we would pull on his collar trying to lead him into the cage, he'd pull back and dig in his paws. It seemed he'd rather choke to death than enter that pen. So here was how we solved the problem: before we left the farm, we held up a Milk-Bone in front of Clem's face. Once we got his attention, we threw it into the pen. Clem bounded into the pen, devoured the biscuit in a few seconds, and, saliva rimming his mouth, turned around to come back out. Of course, in the meantime we had shut the pen door, and thus did Clem stay in one place while we went into town. Every single time we went away, we simply threw a bone into the pen, and, as much as Clem hated being locked up in there, he ran after it.

The point of my story is this: Labrador retrievers, or, at least *our* Lab, may be able to learn that there is a consequence for their actions (being locked in the pen) but, presented with an attractive stimulus (a doggie treat), they cannot suppress the urge to act on their desires. (I'm sure my readers who have cats see this story as yet another laughable example of feline superiority.) Just like Clem, some people cannot prevent themselves from acting on impulses, even when they know negative results may ensue. The inability to inhibit an instinctual reaction is called, in medical parlance, *disinhibition*. And it's the third reason why affairs get the NOD.

I want what I want when I want it

There are lots of cool things that I like. My neighbor has a new power washer in his garage, and I could really use it to clean my gutters. *I'd love to just go over there and take it out of his garage and get to work!* My colleague at work has a new smart phone that does everything but brush his teeth (no, there's no app for that). *Man-oh-man, I would just love to walk over to his desk and take it home so I could use it.* And the other day, at the beach, I really needed a hat and the guy next to me was wearing one with a nice wide brim, perfect to keep the ultraviolet rays off my sensitive ears. *I ought to just grab it off his head, so I can get the sun protection I need.*

In each of these cases, and probably hundreds more each week that I don't even think about, I've got an urge to do something to make me happier or, at the very least, make my life easier. Life is short, right? Shouldn't I just go for it?

It's obvious that the answer is "no." There are lots of reasons why I don't run a red light when I feel like it, take cash out of my patients' pocketbooks when they are distracted, or eat off another customer's table while I wait to be seated at a restaurant. I could be arrested, beaten up, even lose my job, just to name a few possible outcomes. In all of these cases, I maintain a deep understanding that just because I want or need something doesn't mean that I should just take it.

Mind, meet impulse

Most people are able to keep themselves from doing things that will have obvious negative consequences. *After all,* you might be saying, *if someone were to throw a treat in a cage and lock me in, you can bet that I'd never run into that cage again.* But you'd be surprised how, in everyday life, people often fail to prevent bad outcomes for themselves.

Researchers who investigate human behavior have tried to make sense of just why people jump into behaviors that, rationally, they know will spell disaster. Let's take a look at how the human brain is designed. The brain reacts more strongly to something it's never been exposed to before, called *novel stimuli* by psychologists. A new object in your life (whether it's a flat screen television you just bought or the lovely neighbor who just moved in across the street) generates a high release of dopamine (up to four times higher than run-of-the-mill positive experiences) and heightens your sense of pleasure. In ways that only the unconscious mind can appreciate, when you experience an increase in the intensity of emotions, there's a better chance that you might make an impulsive decision. In his book *How We Decide,* science writer Jonah Lehrer describes a built-in flaw in the brain: "emotions . . . tend to overvalue immediate gains (like a new pair of shoes) at the cost of future expenses (high interest rates)." In fact, research shows that just by looking at a photo of an attractive person of the opposite sex, men (but not women) may end up making more short-sighted decisions. For women, it may take more than good looks to generate poor decisions; it often requires emotional stimulation. Remember Mike Torchia, the trainer-turned-Casanova who regularly has affairs with married women? He homes in on the unsuppressed impulses of his clients as they leap headlong into an affair: "I like to make them feel young, mischievous, alive."

Holding on to your horses

One of the greatest challenges confronting all humans is to master the impulse to do something now, so as to prevent having regrets later. When you have your sights on something you really like (or want to avoid something you can't stand), can you stick with your plans to do what's best for you in the long run?

It's not easy to control yearnings. Every year more than a million Americans go bankrupt because they bought things before they had the money to pay for them. People get into car accidents because they get tired of waiting for traffic to clear while pulling out of parking lots onto heavily traveled streets. People walk away from restaurant meals that they looked forward to all week because the hostess informs them they will have a one-hour wait. I don't think I have to list all the things that people (you included) have done, or not done, because they weren't patient enough to wait.

A fascinating study involves a psychologist who sits children in a room with a marshmallow in front of them, just within reach. The researcher tells these children he will be back in fifteen minutes, and, if they can refrain from eating the marshmallow, they will be rewarded with two marshmallow treats. Some children ate the marshmallow immediately; some literally covered their eyes or turned away to prevent themselves from stealing it. Alas, only one-third of the children in the experiment were able to resist the temptation for the entire waiting period.

This book is about infidelity, not marshmallows, and the impulses I am talking about are impulses of adults, not children. But, remarkably, when scientists went back a decade later to find out how these children were faring in life, they found that those who showed very poor impulse control as toddlers carried the same trait into young adulthood. As high school students, they were having more legal and school problems (and lower SAT scores) than were children who were able to delay gratification. By the time they checked in on these people thirty years later, the kids with poor impulse control were more likely to have health and substance abuse issues.

This research suggests that some people are better than others at finding ways to resist impulses and that this trait persists into adulthood. Nearly every day you meet people who may be potential affairmates. It doesn't have to happen at the gym, or at work; it could happen anywhere. If you have an unmet need (and we all do), and an opportunity presents itself (and it will at some point in your life), can you inhibit your impulse to act? In other words, if the door opens up for an affair, do you walk through it? If you have not been able to inhibit the impulse in the past, then there is a high risk that you may not be able to inhibit it in the future. Anyone who has had an affair, to one degree or another, needs to work on improving impulse control to prevent leaping into an act with devastating consequences.

Psychiatric causes of disinhibition

Attention deficit hyperactivity disorder

Wouldn't it be great if people who had problems suppressing their urges could just pop a pill to control disinhibition? It's not so simple. Despite all the medical advances over the past half-century, no medication exists that is indicated specifically to treat disordered impulse control. Yet, there are many emotional or psychiatric problems for which poor impulse control is a symptom. The disorder in which this symptom is most commonly seen is attention deficit hyperactivity disorder (ADHD), which first appears in childhood and is thought to occur in up to 5 percent of people, affecting men more frequently than women. Years ago it was felt that this disorder "disappears" in adulthood because the characteristic ants-in-the-pants hyperactivity seemingly dissipates with age. We now know that residual symptoms of ADHD, including impulsivity, can last through life. Disinhibition that is caused by ADHD can sometimes be controlled with medication. Commonly, physicians will prescribe psychostimulants, such as Ritalin (methylphenidate) or Adderall (amphetamine salts) or other nonstimulant alternatives. Sometimes these medications can work to improve focus and reduce distractibility, thereby helping to protect people from making poor decisions.

Several years ago a woman came to my office seeking help with a postpartum depression. She and her husband had movie-star good looks and a comfortable middle-class life in the suburbs. As she recovered from her depression, she complained to me of marital issues. Although neither she nor her husband had ever strayed, she had felt increasingly frustrated by her husband's apparent inability to sit for more than two minutes and engage in a conversation with her. An interview with her husband led me to realize that he had a history of hyperactivity, problems sitting still, and wandering attention every day since kindergarten. When he started on a small dose of Ritalin, he was able to sit calmly and engage in conversation with his wife for the good part of an hour, without looking away or becoming restless.

But he was not accustomed to sitting still and became bored with his new style of interacting. This is not uncommon—often the inattentiveness of the person with ADHD bothers other people more than it bothers the person with ADHD. Much of the therapy focused on helping him understand the need to keep his symptoms under control not only for his own sake but also for his wife and children.

Substance abuse disorders

Substance abuse disorders are another set of common psychiatric disorders that affect impulse control. Abuse of central nervous system depressants, such as alcohol, barbiturates, heroin, opiates (such as Oxycontin or Percoset), or benzodiazepines (such as Klonopin, Xanax, or Ativan), can result in people acting in ways that they would ordinarily never do when they are not taking these drugs. Almost any drug of abuse, including cocaine, ecstasy, or marijuana, can cause changes in behavior that impede a person's ability to control impulses.

Substance abuse doesn't have to be chronic to be a problem. Specialists in the field recognize that if someone's behavior results in negative consequences (such as a barroom brawl or an arrest for drunk driving), then substance use is risky. One couple I treated was struggling with some difficult financial and work-related marital problems when the husband went on an annual golf trip with his buddies. After golfing, they stopped in at the "nineteenth hole" for drinks, where he struck up a conversation with a married woman who was looking for companionship while on a vacation of her own. The conversation crossed over into an intimate discussion and, with each drink, he developed a stronger attraction. They ended up in bed together, and that one action set off an avalanche of events that led to his wife's filing for divorce. Did he have a need? Yes, he was feeling some need for connection but not enough to propel him to seek an affair. Was there an opportunity? Sure. People who congregate together in casual situations can be a prime source of affair partners, but he had been to other social situations away from his wife and never strayed. Was there disinhibition? Absolutely. This typically in-control and super responsible young man readily admitted that he never would have gone as far as he did without his helping of "liquid courage." This NOD led to a divorce within the year.

Often people don't recognize substance abuse as being a problem. They may rationalize their substance use by saying "everyone does it" or "it doesn't affect me" or by claiming it is a way to deal with underlying anxiety or depression. Whatever the reason, the first step to getting substance abuse under control is to acknowledge that you have a problem. Unfortunately, not many medications have consistently been able to control substance abuse disorders (although advances have been made in the treatment of opiate and alcohol abuse), so individual and group therapies, such as Alcoholics Anonymous (AA), are often necessary.

From the Web: Double Addiction

I am posting this as a way to release guilt and hopefully find some type of therapy in the process. I was married for ten years and have known my soon-to-be ex for fifteen years. I have had various sexual encounters over the course of our relationship. She had found out about them and we have been separated twice, but she had been willing to work at it each time. Once she came back a third time, I did it again. Now we are ending our marriage, and it has devastated me. Yes, I know I am the cause for this and frankly it comes from being addicted to online pornography and marijuana. Those two vices entice me to act inappropriately and put myself in very, very bad situations. I am attempting to get help for my addictions and quit them altogether, and it has been hard. But I know I need that out of my life in order to get back my life.

As for my ex, what devastates me is that she is beautiful, smart, responsible and a loving mother—all of the things anyone would want in a wife—yet I can't seem to get it right. I want her but it seems like only when she doesn't want me. Also in committing these indiscretions I knew that I was risking my marriage yet I subconsciously didn't care. I have seriously injured the person I care the most about, and it hurts me down to the core.

There are times at night I just break down in tears because of the chances
and effort this woman has given over the years. It hurts to know I caused
her to look for happiness somewhere else and yet in some sadistic way try
to look for sympathy from her.

Now our relationship is very businesslike and only involves our children.
She is looking to find new relationships, which I totally understand, and yet I
am hurt by them. No different than what I did to her with my affairs. I am so
ashamed I rarely try to see her face-to-face unless it is absolutely necessary. I
am a pure emotional wreck and I don't know what to do.

Bipolar disorder

Another less common disorder is bipolar disorder (also called manic-
depressive disorder), thought to occur in up to 5 percent of people.
The term literally means "two poles," which I like to think of as a
North Pole and a South Pole. The South Pole consists of depression
(described in the serotonin section of chapter 4), with symptoms of
low mood, lack of energy, poor sleep, and even suicidal thoughts.
While depression can include symptoms of anxiety or agitation, it
usually results in social withdrawal, so there may be less risk of affairs.
(Occasionally, people with depression seek out sex as a way of feeling
better, but this isn't usually seen as an impulse control problem.)

When individuals with bipolar disorder experience the North
Pole—called mania—they are the opposite of depressed. People with
manic episodes often have elevated mood and even delusions of gran-
diosity—with ideas that they have millions of dollars stashed away or
that they have written all the songs that Katy Perry performs. In the
midst of a mania, they may have racing thoughts, irritability, distractibility, and impulsivity and engage in reckless and dangerous activities
without regard to consequences. It's easy to see how someone in this
situation could end up in bed with someone who they would never
otherwise be with.

If you see your mate's moods going up and down, or you yourself
have problems controlling impulses, can bipolar disorder explain your
relationship problems? Psychiatrists are increasingly labeling disinhibited moody individuals as being "bipolar," but true bipolar disorder

is not simply a syndrome where people have tendencies toward poor decision making and out-of-control behavior. Yes, it is an illness of changing moods, but these changes *don't* happen minute-to-minute or even day-to-day. Bipolar is the presence of mental state in which behaviors *uncharacteristic* of that person emerge. In other words, someone who would not normally be hyperactive, irritable, or talkative begins to act in this revved up way and continues to do so for many days in a row (to the point where he or she won't need to sleep because of excessive energy). When people with true bipolar disorder have a manic episode, they are quite disinhibited, often have a higher sex drive, and may be particularly at risk for affairs. Many medications have been shown to effectively prevent or control mania.

Other psychiatric causes

Individuals who have certain personality disorders, such as borderline, antisocial, or histrionic disorders and some forms of narcissistic personality disorder can also have severe disinhibition. These complicated psychiatric illnesses are thought to develop early in a person's life and reflect maladaptive ways of coping with stress and other people. Often people don't know they have these disorders and tend to put the blame on others for a long string of relationship and work problems.

Personality disorders cannot be easily managed with medications, and in some cases, such as antisocial personality (see chapter 4), even psychotherapy is unlikely to help. Generally, though, under care of a qualified treatment team, including a psychiatrist and talk therapist, people who have personality disorders can minimize their symptoms and experience genuine improvement in their quality of life.

Brain damage or other brain illnesses

Another common cause of disinhibition is brain damage, which can result from skiing accidents, falls, or motorcycle crashes—indeed, any head injury is a big risk factor for brain damage. But many people (men more than women) have subtler brain injury that can lead to an impaired control of impulses. Early childhood deprivation or dietary problems (or exposure to lead or other toxins) can cause impaired brain control. As individuals age, they are also at risk for changes in behavior based not on brain damage that is not from outside the body but from within. Small strokes (blockage or breakage of blood vessels supplying the brain) or degenerative illnesses (such as Alzheimer disease or frontal lobe dementia) may affect parts of the brain that suppress impulses. Earlier in the chapter, I mentioned wishing to take a power washer out of my neighbor's garage or to eat off of another restaurant patron's plate. Some people with brain damage would do these things without consideration of why other people would object. Some people with moderate to advanced cases of these degenerative disorders make lewd gestures or sexual advances without regard to their marital vows. While some pharmacological interventions can improve memory and daily functioning of people who have some dementias, these disinhibited behaviors are not easily managed through medications.

Getting control of your impulses

If you have any of these psychiatric disorders (and some people have a combination of them), that doesn't mean that you have an excuse to have an affair. If medication helps, then you have the responsibility to take it; if psychotherapy is prescribed, then you must make a commitment to attend sessions. In the most severe cases of these disorders, individuals may not be competent to forge a marriage contract. But otherwise I strongly believe that capable individuals who make the choice to wed should be held responsible for doing whatever it takes to keep their vows.

If you are married to someone who has a problem inhibiting impulses, you may feel overwhelmed at times. But more than likely (unless your partner suffered brain damage or a dementia after you married) your partner's wildness, irreverence, and spontaneity were among the qualities that most appealed to you when you chose to marry. You may have enjoyed some of the freedom that comes along with this personality type. Now that you are married, though, you have a right to anticipate a modicum of predictability in your life. At the very least, you should expect that your partner will be faithful.

Both partners must make changes to minimize the impact of disinhibition on the marriage.

This list is for the married person who has not been able to suppress his or her impulses:

1 Reduce opportunities.
  a. Stay away from single individuals or married people who are "playing the field."
  b. Don't hang with friends who are having affairs or who support infidelity in any way.
  c. Stop using any alcohol or drugs, which further reduce impulses.

2 Think things through. Once you recognize that impulsivity has led to trouble in your life, you can learn new habits for managing your desires.
  a. Keep a journal to record your thoughts in different situations. This will force you to write things down and think things through before you act. Even if you don't have pad and paper or computer on hand, there are "notepad" functions in most cell phones, so you can still stop to take note of what you are thinking. In other words, "check in" with yourself.
  b. Seek consultation before acting. If you're not sure what direction to take, look for someone you can discuss the situation with. One of the first persons you should talk to is your spouse. For instance, if you are invited to happy hour after work, before you say yes, consult with your partner to ask whether it's a good idea.
  c. Play the "what if?" game. People who are impulsive are prone to be excessively confident about outcomes, believing things such as "no one will find out," "nothing bad will happen from this," or "I can control myself in any situation." Instead of accepting the most optimistic outlook, think about what would happen if things go wrong. One single male medical

student I treated started flirting with a married nurse while doing his emergency room rotation. When an invitation was extended to have an affair, he thought about what would happen if her husband found out and came after him with a gun. It stopped the affair cold! When you look at the worst-case scenario, it may prevent you from taking that next disastrous step.

3   Seek professional help. A thorough assessment of your emotional state can help you understand if there are any psychiatric or psychological reasons that could be making it hard for you to delay gratification. Your therapist can help you form a plan to overcome your problems and hold you accountable for your success in achieving your goals.

4   Get control of your brainwaves. Medical research conducted over the course of thirty years has shown that regular meditation can reduce stress, calm the mind, and improve cognitive processes (not to mention helping to treat headache and reducing blood pressure). Any kind of commitment to non-drug-induced relaxation, prayer, yoga, or aerobic exercise can help you improve your brain functioning. Having a relaxed brain can help you think through decisions better.

This list is for the person whose life partner is impulsive:

1   Don't nag or whine. Living with a reckless person can be very frustrating, but people don't change because they are nagged. You know that already. You can avoid badgering your partner, if, rather than critiquing him or her on the spot, you sit down together when things aren't stressed, and both reach an agreement that the impetuousness is a problem. If an affair has already happened, make a plan moving forward. Decide jointly that if you feel that an impulsive decision is being made, you will have a prearranged signal that a boundary is being crossed. It can be a

hand sign (such as a capital *T*), putting on an ugly tie-die shirt, or even sending a friendly command via text message (such as "Hold on there, Cowboy!"). These signals should be designed to make a clear point while eliminating the harsh words and arguments that often accompany your disapproval.

2 Once you and your partner have made the decision to follow this protocol, it's in your partner's hand what happens once the signal is received. Your partner can choose to stop and talk with you about your concerns or ignore you altogether. He or she is an adult, and you can't make those choices for him or her. The important point here is that you made your apprehension known without nagging or fighting. If the behavior does not change (and your partner forges ahead despite your signal), in all probability he or she would not have changed the behavior even if you had nagged or whined.

3 Offer healthy alternatives. If your partner calls you asking permission to sail with his boss on a boat named *Risky Business*, or she wants to spend a weekend in Las Vegas with her single girlfriends, it helps to be able to offer an alternative, less precarious, activity. Think of things that can be equally exciting and fun, and can involve you as a couple, or will allow the partner to spend time with people who may be a good influence.

4 Be patient and supportive. In most cases your mate has always been disinhibited; it's not a trait he or she can grow out of in a few weeks or months. In some cases, the poor impulse control may come on the heels of a life-changing event (such as the death of a parent) or a "midlife crisis." Offer support, and ally with your mate's desire to have things get better. People respond to positive reinforcement, so letting your partner know (either with words, gifts, or physical touch) that you appreciate his or her efforts will improve motivation for improvement. (I'll address that further in chapter 11.)

5 Loosen up! I'll bet your partner says this to you all the time.
   And if you're like most of my patients in this situation, you say
   to yourself, "Someone has to be the responsible one here!" But
   (1) you won't become irresponsible if you relax on some issues
   and (2) if you always play the responsible role, than your partner
   must figure, "Someone has to be the irresponsible one around
   here!" Anyway, it's natural to want to correct for one person's
   extreme behavior by becoming extreme in the other direction. But if your spouse enjoys spontaneity, small changes in
   your behavior can make him more attracted to your newfound
   spunkiness and may make other options less attractive.

6 Support efforts to change. If your partner has made alterations in
   health or behavior to improve his impulsivity—such as meditation, AA meetings, religious activities, or exercise—offer to
   join with him or her in the activity. Permanent change is always
   easier when it is done with the support and companionship of
   loved ones.

❧ THE NEXT STEP

We live a life full of needs, we exist in a world full of opportunities,
and on a daily basis we struggle against disinhibition of impulses. It
takes courage, control, and sometimes luck to keep clear of the NOD
of affairs. But when an affair does hit, you've got to be prepared to
make some changes in your life and in your relationship. We'll talk
about that in the next chapter.

6

Affair Exposed, Now What?

Do you know how to open a bag of potato chips? Sure! You've done it hundreds of times. Now, do you know how to open the release valve on the Space Shuttle?

Knowing how to do things is easy when you've confronted them over and over. But if you have never come across a challenge before—like getting out of a spaceship—you can't be expected to know how to manage it. Following the revelation of an affair, many couples make a conscious decision to stay together as they try to move forward past a hurtful situation. Because they rarely, or never, had to confront this situation before, they may not know the best course of action to take. They will almost certainly take some missteps along the way. Affairs don't come with instructions in dealing with the aftermath. If ever any endeavor in human interaction needed an instruction booklet, however, it would be dealing with infidelity.

✣ POSTAFFAIR INSTRUCTIONS

In my years of helping couples with infidelity, I saw over and over again that couples did not know how to go forward. For example, what is the best way to ask your partner about an affair? How should a spouse respond to those questions? What kind of contact, if any, should the spouse have with the third person involved? I wrote this "postaffair instruction book" because I have seen in my patients that there is a right way and a wrong way to go about recovering from an affair. Once you know the four steps to take in the recovery process, you can start moving forward.

Of course the specifics of every affair vary greatly. Despite these different details (such as how the affair happened, how many affairs, who was involved, how long the deceit lasted, how the partner found out, and whether the affair is still going on), the general four steps apply. Like any other instruction book, this one recommends completing the first step before moving on to the next one. That is the best way to reach your objective.

✣ STEP 1: END THE AFFAIR

This may seem obvious and sensible, but you'd be surprised how often this most critical of healing steps is overlooked. I meet with many couples where the man or woman is still maintaining some contact with the person he or she had the affair with. If you're in that situation yourself, you may be confused about how, and why, your partner would still choose to hurt you by keeping the affair going.

I understand your pain, and I don't support your spouse having continued contact with the person he or she was having an affair with. But before you and I together simply stare in disbelief at your mate, I think it's worth taking a few minutes to figure out how he or she sees things. I want you to understand that what can be so apparent to you and me may not be so obvious to your mate.

Many people who have had an affair are in a state of confusion. Priorities, values, goals, needs all get mixed up when an affair has started. So it may not be crystal clear to your partner why the affair should end. Yes, you heard me right: your partner may not understand that the affair has to stop. You need to appreciate why it's not sinking in to him or her that it does have to stop.

Why contact continues

Here are the reasons a spouse may give for keeping alive the relationship with the third party:

1   "I shouldn't deny myself the pleasures that I'm getting out of the relationship; not only is the sex appealing, but I like the special way I feel when I'm with this person. It's a better feeling than what I get in my marriage. Don't I deserve to feel good?"

2   "I have found my soul mate. This person I'm having an affair with is very special, and I don't think I'll find someone like him (or her) again if I break up this relationship. I don't want to give up a connection that feels even more special than my marriage."

3   "I feel a duty to this other person, and it's disrespectful and hurtful for me to throw him (or her) out to the curb because we are having marriage problems; it's not his (or her) fault that our marriage is in trouble."

4   "I wasn't strong enough (or smart enough, or skilled enough) to fix the mess that our marriage was in, and I'm not strong/smart/ skilled enough to fix *this* mess."

In the world of a flame addict, options aren't clear. The idea of giving up the pursuit of the flame may generate panic. This third person fills a void, and to give up that person not only removes your obsessive ideal but takes away a cushion between you and your spouse. No paramour—nowhere to hide. From your mate or from yourself.

If you are having an affair and you aren't ready to cast aside your lover, I understand. But I don't agree. I'd like to explain why keeping another person in your life, or in the wings, will severely impede any chance at getting your marriage back on track.

Why the contact should stop

1. *If the affair continues . . .* your partner will seem less desirable. Think about all the times you've seen your mate first thing in the morning, hair toussled and breath smelling like a pair of old socks. Think about all the disagreements you've had with your partner about money, children, housework, or in-laws (not to mention sex). Day in and day out, you face a lot of unpleasant realities about life with your mate. There's no way your spouse can compete with someone who is always well-groomed and fresh-smelling when you see him or her, who doesn't argue with you, who you don't have to balance checkbooks with or fight over whose family's house you're going to for Christmas. On top of which, the person you're having an affair with has a great sexual appetite! He or she is on for you all the time (just the way you and your spouse were for each other when you first met); face it, your spouse just can't keep up that same standard. In comparison, you'll see your partner as the one who needs to get dumped. Holding your partner up to that standard isn't fair.

2. *If the affair continues . . .* there will be less time for your partner and you to solve problems together. I wish I could tell you that happy marriages never have arguments. I'd be lying. But I can tell you that if you've had some tough spells with your mate, it takes time to work through them. In families where infidelity is *not* an issue, there is still plenty of conflict. Many disagreements can take place over several hours or days. Let's say, for example, a wife makes a harsh comment toward her hubby, something like: "You're the only man I know who has to consult his smart phone to buy a loaf of bread!" A husband may have hurt feelings and accuse his wife of being rude. The wife may get defensive, saying, "I was just joking. You're just too thin skinned!"

Later that day, she may apologize, but he may hold a grudge. Still later on, he may offer an olive branch, and she may or may not accept. Yes, it's one of those fights that no one can recall a week later, but when it's going on, it's not pleasant, and, like two boxers in a ring, a man and wife must invest the time and energy to duke it out, until they can finally come to some resolution.

Solving problems doesn't have to be about having a fight. Sometimes a decision as simple as "Where should we go for dinner?" requires thought and discussion. Being in the same place at the same time smoothes the way for good decision making.

When you are spending time with, e-mailing, texting, or otherwise in communication with someone outside your home, you are taken away from being with your family. If you put your attention on a person outside your marriage during a time when you and your spouse disagree about something, you may walk away before any resolution is reached—before each of you can go through the stressful but necessary steps of patching things up and moving on. You may be left with the false conclusion that you and your mate never agree on anything, when, in reality, you ran away before agreement was possible.

If you are going to work together on solving problems, you have to be fully in the marriage.

3. *If the affair continues . . .* there will be less time for you and your partner to share positive times together. Think about watching a baseball game. Pitch after pitch, swing after swing, sometimes whole hours can go by before anything significant happens. Then, in what seems like an instant, there's a man on second and your favorite steroid-juiced homerun king is up to bat. And there's only one out. Now things get good! Baseball isn't a thrilling game because something is always going on; baseball is a thrilling game because something exciting could always happen. It's a lot of waiting around, and then something amazing happens.

Marriage is a lot like baseball. Sometimes it's mundane. But thrilling things can happen in marriage at any time, if you're there to experience them. When you're involved with someone else, you may mistakenly believe that your marriage is boring or, worse, destructive. Escaping into another relationship interrupts the ebb and flow of marriage, so that you never really experience the exciting times that would be in store for you if you hung around.

Special moments, although not every minute of every day, spring up if you look for them. You stop looking when something (or someone) else has got your attention.

4. *If the affair continues* . . . a back door will be propped open. When you know there's an easy way out of a problem, it's natural to take it. If you know that you can walk away from difficulties you are having with your mate, you won't be nearly so creative about how fix the problem. If, however, you know there's no way out, you'll discover unknown resources, hidden talents, flashes of insight, or just plain gumption that you never knew you had. That's a by-product of being forced to put something right. Having another lover you can turn to when you are having marital problems robs you of your ability to create or persevere. If you allow him or her to stay in your life, you might, despite your best intentions, end up doing what comes naturally and exit your marriage out the still-open door.

♣ STEP 2: SEVER THE CONNECTION

Charlene and Phil are a couple I treated many years ago. They described a brief affair that Charlene had had when she attended her twentieth high school reunion. When the affair came out, they decided to come see me for therapy together because they wanted to save the marriage. I explained to them just what I explained to you. Stop the affair! Charlene readily agreed. The guy lived two states over, so she didn't anticipate that it would continue anyway. The following week the three of us met for our session. I was full of hope that the couple was ready to begin the healing process.

In that session, Charlene proudly announced that the affair had ended. Phil, however, did not seem so pleased. While it was true that

Charlene sent a very clear e-mail (which Phil had read in advance) saying "adios" to her paramour, she still continued to be his friend and chat with him on Facebook. "Charlene . . ." I murmured, "Maybe there was something I forgot to tell you. When I say break things off with him, I mean break everything off with him. You must end *all* communications. That's key to healing your marriage." Charlene hasn't been in touch with the guy since.

This is another example of how people simply don't know the rules about infidelity. I don't think Charlene was stupid, and I don't think she was intentionally being cruel, she just did what she would do in any normal relationship when she didn't hate someone: she kept up a friendship but on a different level. Charlene had to learn that cutting ties with her high school sweetheart is a must.

I've learned my lesson as a therapist also. Now, whenever I help people to see that the affair must end, I also help them understand that all communication with that person must end.

There are many variations on "continued contact":

- Ongoing sexual contact (although, in this case, it's pretty clear that even Rule #1 wasn't followed, so is there much hope for Rule #2?)
- Maintaining telephone or Internet contact
- Exchanging mail or text greetings (like birthday wishes)
- Spending time together at work
- Silent contact; in other words, ending the affair, but agreeing that they will each "wait in the wings" in case their marriages don't work out

The rationale for Step #2 is no different from that of Step #1: saving a marriage requires the full attention of both partners. If you're the victim of infidelity, this may seem like a no-brainer, but if you're the one who has had a relationship outside of marriage, you may find this objectionable. In fact, there is no step in recovering from an affair that is more difficult to take than severing the connection.

There are many reasons why the communication between a person who has had an affair and his or her affair mate continues. I'll share here some of the reasons. I'll save the surprising most common reason for last.

Scenario 1: The unfaithful partner wants the affair to continue or is on the fence about whether to still see this person

If your partner cheated on you and now refuses to halt contact, his or her reasons may just seem like pathetic excuses. But, if you look at it from your spouse's point of view, each of these reasons makes sense in its own way. However, for every "reason" to keep contact with an ex-affair mate, there are many more reasons why the contact must end.

From the Web: She Wants to Explore

My wife recently came to me and told me she is having an affair with her female boss. I still love her very much and do not want a divorce, but she refuses to end the affair. She has reawakened passion with this other woman and wants to keep exploring that. She won't commit to saving our marriage and won't stop the affair, but she doesn't want to lose what we have either.

Nathan, married nine years

Another reason your partner may refrain from shutting down lines of communication is because maintaining contact keeps the fires of passion burning. In this case, failure to follow through with Step #2 really reflects an inability to complete the first step: ending the affair. So I'll remind you once more: Moving ahead in your marriage requires the unfaithful partner to extinguish those passionate fires, and that means cutting off all fuel for the flame.

Scenario 2: The partner having the affair lacks the technical know-how to block messages or restrict phone calls

Even someone who sincerely wants the affair to end may not be sophisticated in the world of electronic communication. Some of my clients really did not know how to block calls on their phone or remove friends from Internet or Facebook lists. Occasionally this ignorance is intentional, reflecting mixed feelings about shutting down communication. Like the teenager who "doesn't know" how to run the washing machine (so he can still have his parents do the laundry) but can be taught easily, the man or woman who claims to be a computer dunce can learn how to shut down electronic communications. Start with a phone call to your cell phone or Internet provider. It may take a few calls and e-mails after that, but eventually, together, you can put a stranglehold on these electronic messages.

From the Web: He Continues to Call and Write

I never thought that I could be one of "those women," the kind of woman who would date a married man. I fell into it and was led to believe he was separated from his wife; by the time he told me the truth, I had already fallen in love. I tried several times to get out of it but was drawn back in by my own naive stupidity. He promised me the world; he wrote me poetry; he met my mom (and she liked him), etc. I thought we would be together forever, just as soon as he got out of his "situation." His wife found out about me. She confronted him; then, she started calling me. I lied to her. She quoted Bible verses and called me a harlot (who uses that word?). She was right, I was wrong, but so was he. He assured me that they were working out the arrangements to end their marriage. She continued to harass me at work, at home, everywhere. The thing that never made sense to me is that she kept only blaming me and kept forgiving him. So, finally, I had enough, and I told him I was tired of feeling bad all the time, tired of being afraid to answer my phone, tired of not being able to go out in public, just tired. So, I broke up. *Over a year later, he continues to call and write and leave little presents at my house.* I was told that they are still together and that six months ago they renewed their vows. If you write this book, maybe you can explain the *why* of all this? I'd love to read it.

—Amanda, 36, married once previously

Scenario 3: The affair partner works with the person he or she was cheating with and feels unable to scale back interactions

Workplace affairs are problematic, because it's not easy to draw a line between necessary work interactions and communication that could harm your marriage. In many cases the constant work contact between two people who are trying to end an affair is just overwhelming. In these cases, ending communication may mean making major changes to your job. This may seem like a drastic step. It *is* a drastic step. But too many people dismiss this possibility because they don't want to change anything at work. Here's the deal: if you work every day with and sit in a chair next to (or ride in a car next to or key data next to) the person you are trying to end an affair with, then it will be virtually impossible to cut out communication, and that may destroy your marriage. At Alcoholics Anonymous, one of the caveats of successful sobriety is staying away from bars. There's a saying to the effect: "If you hang out at a barbershop, eventually you'll get your hair cut." You may think that you can resist the attraction of the flame, but it is not something that willpower alone can resist.

Making major changes at your place of employment doesn't mean you have to quit your job, although don't eliminate it from the range of possibilities. Consider a transfer to a different building or different floor within the building. Think about changing your schedule, so you are no longer there at the same time as the other person. This may mean a sit-down with your boss or manager, and it may mean disclosing the workplace affair. (Before going to your boss, be sure to determine that such a disclosure won't get you fired. Many human resources policies encourage their employees to be open about workplace relationships. After all, more than anyone, your employer wants you to stay focused on your work.) In some cases, it may take some negotiating with the person you had an affair with. Find out whether he or she would change jobs. But, in all probability, since you're the one with the most to lose, you'll have to be the one making changes.

Solving the problem of a workplace affair takes creativity on the part of husband and wife. It may also require sacrifices that you didn't anticipate when you started to work on healing your relationship. Indeed, this sacrifice may ultimately include the possibility of moving to a new job, or even a new town, in order to completely shut down communication.

From the Web: Caught in the Trap

I got caught in the trap of an emotional affair in my past and repented immensely and have *never* again strayed from my wife either in mind, spirit, or body. We were married five years before I stepped out and finally woke up to the error of my ways and asked for forgiveness and followed up with actions for the past eight years. Technology is a dangerous tool for access to anyone around the globe. As my work needs me to use a computer, I struggle with even having one for work and the kids. But I know that the horrible pain and suffering I caused my wife can *never* happen again. I even avoid female coworkers so as not to damage my relationship with my wife. As much as I would like a woman's perspective on situations in the marriage, I can't go down that road. It may start off as innocent, but, as soon as the feelings of understanding between a husband and a woman coworker start, the path leads to danger.

Scenario 4: The affair partner is friend or family of the spouse

Of all of the infidelity issues I come up against, I think the most difficult is when an affair happens between a spouse and an in-law. The level of betrayal, sky-high with any affair, is extraordinarily so when the person you marry sleeps with a person in your wedding party. I wish that pulling away from contact could be as simple as changing jobs or phone numbers, but the links to family are difficult to break. The bottom line is this: as much as possible, avoid contact with the family member who participated in damaging your marriage. If your family member or best friend cheated with your spouse, your best bet is to refuse phone calls or messages requesting "an opportunity to explain" or apologies until you and your spouse are able to work on your own issues. If you were the one who cheated with your in-law, you must agree to make whatever changes are necessary in your routines, vacations, and holiday schedules so you have no contact with that person. Some couples can eventually reintegrate themselves back into the family; some cannot. The most powerful choice you and your spouse can make is to decide to join together as a "first family" and to make the preservation of your relationship a priority.

The most common reason for not severing the connection
If you've been the victim of a spouse cheating on you, you may be stunned by what I'm about to tell you. What I've learned from my patients is that the most common reason someone won't stop talking to the person they had an affair with is . . . it's rude.

If you have been the victim of an affair and are wondering why your mate has not built a fifty-foot brick wall between himself or herself and "*that* person," it may come down to something as mundane as your partner not wanting to display bad manners. Rationally, you have every right to be outraged by this revelation. If anyone was rude to anyone, it was your mate who offended you! Yes, but . . .

In most cultures, people are very good at ending a relationship when they feel hurt or offended. I see this all time. A daughter forgets a father's birthday and Dad writes her out of the will; one neighbor calls the cops on another for his barking dog and they never speak again; or the accountant messes up on your income taxes and you delete her number from your contacts. When someone does something to screw with us, most of us are willing to shut down all contact.

But we are taught not to be rude to people who have done nothing to upset or offend us. I understand that the person *cheated on* has every reason to feel animosity toward the third party. However, in the eyes of the cheating spouse, the third party was courteous, discreet, and, let's face it, very giving. Most people are not very good at shutting down relations with people they like, including an affair mate.

A neighborly affair
Dawn is a good example of such a person. Soon after her seventh anniversary with her husband, Khalil, the couple sought consultation with me. Khalil had discovered that she was having an affair with a divorced father, Brian, who lived across the street from them. The friendship began innocently enough, as Dawn and Brian had stood by the school bus stop morning and afternoon attending to their young sons. After more than a year, they decided to go for lunch together. Afterward, they spent more and more time together, and Khalil knew nothing of the meetings.

Dawn's life with her husband was stable but not all that exciting, and Khalil admits, "There are definitely things I should have done differently." But the affair with Brian excited Dawn. While he didn't lavish her with gifts, he gave her a lot of attention. Sometimes they would have their kids meet for a play date while Khalil was at work, using that as a chance to sneak off into the bedroom. After six months, Khalil began to recognize the signs of an affair and asked Dawn about it. She admitted to it immediately.

Khalil and Dawn had much soul-searching to do about the quality of their relationship, and they also needed to answer some fundamental questions about whether they wanted to work on their marriage. But, now, right now, they wanted to know what to do next.

You should know by now I advised Step #1, and Dawn was on board with ending the affair: "I didn't invest all these years with Khalil for nothing. I want a relationship with the man I married, not our neighbor." But, when it came to my suggestion that Dawn break off communication with Brian, that was a different matter. "I can't do that! After all, he lives across the street. He's a nice guy, and he's been through enough trauma with his ex-wife. I couldn't just shut him out."

I use this case to illustrate how common it is for well-meaning people to falter when it comes down to doing what they have to do for the sake of the marriage. At first Khalil was incredulous, but with my help, he was able to appreciate that Dawn's response was natural and wasn't meant as an offense to him. By the time the couple had returned the following week, the issue was settled. Khalil himself had confronted Brian, and, with tempered rage, told him to totally and completely stay away from his wife. (Unlike Dawn, Khalil had every reason to feel miffed by Brian, so it was easy for him to close a door on him.) Dawn supported Khalil's assertive stance. In fact, she was impressed with it, and she told me she felt protected and comforted by Khalil.

To this day, all three neighbors see each other from time to time, and they nod and wave appropriately, but all but essential communication between Dawn and Brian has ceased. Dawn and Khalil have been able to strengthen their marriage without outside interference.

Their story helps to illustrate one of the most important concepts of this book: If you are involved in an affair and feel uncomfortable ending the relationship, remember: Your mate (not your lover) is the one you made a promise to. You owe nothing to this other person. Your obligation is to your spouse. Period.

Breaking it off
How to say good-bye
For Khalil and Dawn, the communication ended when Khalil confronted Brian. That's one way to end an affair and not a bad one at that, as long as it's done civilly. You and your mate can work together in a number of ways to put the brakes on the extramarital affair. You need to follow a few essential guidelines:

- The message must be absolutely clear.
- You should leave no open doors for a future relationship.
- When possible, your mate should be witness to the breakup.
- Any communication in response to the breakup must be shared with your partner.

When people are having affairs, they find all kinds of ways of communicating. Now that you've decided to break it off, any form of communication can be used. People can break off relationships through phone, online chat or e-mail, text, mail, or in person. Each has its pros and cons. When you send an e-mail or write a letter, it has the benefit of being a complete and reproducible representation of your intention to move on. At that moment, and from that moment on, you, your mate, and even the person you had an affair with will know exactly where you stand.

Phoning or instant messaging may also work, but these modes of communication require more spontaneity than constructing an e-mail or letter and also involve some back and forth, which, unless you have a prepared speech in mind, can throw you off your message. The conversation of a phone call, unless recorded, will not last beyond the moment you push the "end" button. Like e-mails, instant messaging can be copied and stored, so your words can last well past clicking off the chat site. Because they tend to be unstructured, though, there may be more room for mistakes. You should leave no ambiguity when ending an affair. I recommend that if you do use instant messaging or phone call, you first write out what you mean to say, so you are not left tongue-tied during this very important interaction.

Here is an example of a message that is short but will get the point across in an e-mail or text—or even a tweet!

My spouse is writing this w/ me. I can't see you again. I need to work on my marriage. Please don't contact me. Good luck. Don't contact me.

As you can see from this example, "Don't contact me" is stated twice, since the instinct of anyone receiving this communication would be to attempt to get in touch with its author. In fact, when you ask a lover to stay away, your request may trigger an obsession stronger than ever. It's like telling a child, "Don't touch that freshly baked cookie." You become almost irresistible when you break off the affair; that's the nature of a flame addiction.

When you do break it off, you must make it absolutely clear that contact must cease. This is extremely reassuring to your spouse. You have no control over whether or not your newly declared ex will honor your request for space. But you do have control over what to do when he or she attempts to reconnect with you.

When the phone rings

At some point your ex will try to get in touch with you. These days, it's not likely to be a phone call; it's probably going to be a text, an e-mail, or a message on Facebook. The message you get may be a desperate call for you to return, it may be a threat of suicide, or it may carry an implication of threat to harm your family. If there is any threat, you must take steps to protect your ex's life or the safety of your family. That's important to do, but you must do it without contacting your ex. If you know of a family member or mutual friend who can intervene, reach out to that person. If you think you or your family may be at risk, then you must call the police and, if necessary, get a restraining order.

In most cases, you will not get extreme and worrisome threats. Instead, you will probably get a lighthearted text saying something like, "Just wanted to say Hey!" "Miss you!" or "You'll never guess who I ran into!" These are all bids for your attention.

Ignore them. Do not answer. And whenever such communication occurs, tell your partner.

The partner's job

If you've had an affair, you're reading this chapter realizing that I've loaded a lot on you. I hope you follow my advice. Now I shift my focus to the member of the partnership who has not strayed, for that person also has some work to do.

First, when your mate has to make that call to end the affair, you should be by his or her side. You can help construct a breakup letter or suggest things to say online. I understand that you are devastated by the events of the affair, but in this endeavor, you must be your mate's cheerleader and must encourage every step of the breakup.

You may be wondering, *Why should I help in the breakup? I wasn't the one who started the whole thing!* It's a legitimate question, but remember that this is a difficult and confusing time for your mate also. Studies tell us that people grow closer to those who stand by them when they go through traumatic experiences. Just by being with your mate during tough times, you'll improve the bond you have with each other.

Another one of your tasks, tough as it might be, is to express appreciation and encouragement whenever your mate tells you that the ex tried to get in touch with him or her. You may be irritated by this: after all, you reason, perhaps your spouse is trying to encourage these communications in some way, or maybe there was a small opening left when he or she called off the affair. Finding out about *yet another* correspondence may feel to you like it is reopening the wound and keeping you from ever healing. But your partner has no control over whether or not the ex tries to make contact again. Yes, he or she has control over a Facebook page and a chat list. And you two had better agree on shutting them down. But when a call, text, or e-mail arrives, don't assume it was encouraged. Moreover, each time the cell phone buzzes or the inbox tells you you've got mail, your mate has a choice—to tell you or not. When a message does arrive, it's not de facto evidence that your mate is up to no good.

On the receiving end

One couple I treated, Claire and Evan, are a good example of the importance of sharing information. This couple had just gotten remarried after breaking up five years earlier from a sexual affair of Evan's. Now they were just getting over Evan's emotional affair with Alexis, a different woman, which he had broken off four months before. Then, around Evan's forty-fifth birthday, he got a quick e-mail from Alexis, saying, not surprisingly, "Happy Birthday." Evan did not reply, and he immediately told Claire about the e-mail. According to Evan (and Claire agreed): "Claire lost it." At first she became despondent, but soon it bubbled up into rage. Claire was angry with Alexis for her brazen effort to reestablish a connection with Evan. She didn't tell Alexis all this, of course; she ranted at Evan. Evan endured several hours of hostility and accusations until he successfully reassured Claire that there was nothing going on.

The waters grew still for a while, and about three months later Alexis e-mailed Evan with some "news" about a new job she landed in another city. Evan understood he was supposed to tell Claire immediately, but he confessed to me he did not: "Scott, I knew she was just about to get on a flight to a business conference, and I didn't want to shake her up before she was due to give a big talk. If she found out Alexis e-mailed me, she'd blow her top! The news would spoil her mood, probably ruin her flight, and heaven knows what would happen to her lecture. I thought I would wait until after the lecture and let her know."

At the same time that this was going on in Evan's mind, here's what was going on in Claire's mind: "I don't trust him." Years of affairs and near-affairs resulted in her regularly checking up on his correspondence—with Evan's approval. (We'll talk about the issue of transparency in the next section of this chapter.) Claire entered the boarding area for her flight, and, with a half-hour to spare, began to check Evan's e-mails. She was outraged when she saw the opened e-mail from Alexis. "Why hadn't Evan called to tell me?" she asked herself, "That was the deal."

Perhaps Evan didn't call Claire because he had all kinds of nefarious ideas about arranging a hook-up with Alexis, but, frankly, I doubt it. Here's what I think happened: Over the weeks and months of Claire's anger and suspiciousness at her husband, she trained Evan to avoid any discussion of any contact with any woman. The intensity of Claire's reaction was overwhelming to Evan, and he would do anything to avoid it. In essence, Claire had taught Evan *not* to tell her what's going on.

Claire and Evan joined me for a visit the following week. When Claire was able to understand how her actions were working against what she desired, she made a real effort to change. The three of us discussed the concept of the "attractive person" (see chapter 1), and Claire agreed that if Evan had contact with any attractive woman (particularly Alexis), Evan would e-mail her immediately. That would give her time to process her own emotional reaction and give a measured, not an emotional, response. She then was permitted to answer Evan's e-mail with positive responses only, such as, "Thanks for telling me," "I appreciate your letting me know," or "I'm glad that you let me in on this. It helps a lot." When Evan and Claire return to the same room, they can then talk together about what ought to be done. By reinforcing Evan's openness, rather than punishing him, she has found that he is more likely to keep her in the loop, and both of them benefit.

❧ STEP 3: CREATE A SEE-THROUGH MARRIAGE

Unveiling an affair is a huge step. Letting go of the object of the affair and focusing back on the marriage speaks volumes about the person who committed infidelity. Such actions are a relief to the spouse who was cheated on and go quite a way toward reestablishing trust. But not all the way. For this person, rebuilding trust takes time. And the partners who committed infidelity must help them do that in every way possible. One necessary ingredient in this process is transparency.

Transparency 101

Simply put, transparency requires that if you have committed adultery, then your partner must be able to have access to all interactions you have with other people. Your Facebook, Google+, and other social networking interactions must be in full view of your spouse. That also means that your cell phone records for calls and texts are also accessible to your husband or wife. Your bank account and credit card information: fully viewable by all. In addition, the password to your e-mail—all your e-mail accounts—are known by your partner. If you have the technological knowhow, it means keeping your GPS on your phone active and allowing your mate to track your whereabouts. Transparency requires the breaking down, and the continued elimination, of all barriers between you and your mate when it involves the outside world.

Does this seem extreme? Many people are shocked at my suggestion that the person who had an affair, in order to set things right, must lose all right to privacy. I get that; it's a big pill to swallow in a world where passwords are a prerequisite to doing something as simple as checking a voice mail. But the model of transparency is one whose beginnings predate electronic communications.

Think about life forty years ago when cell phones did not exist and the only form of electronic communication was Morse code. (Okay, I exaggerate.) Back then, we relied on the postman for communication. Now, picture a delivery coming to the mailbox and seeing your mate run out to the box, quickly sort through the letters, snatch up an envelope or two and disappear to a hidden alcove. Your mate returns five minutes later and—surprise!—the letters are no longer in hand. Your mate mumbles some excuse about losing them or doing everyone a favor by tearing up the "junk mail." I think it's pretty clear anyone who would act that way would heighten the spouse's suspicion. Most of us would agree that such behavior forty years ago, or even today, would be wrong. Well, how is that different from keeping an e-mail password hidden from your mate? It isn't.

Phones, same deal. Forty years ago, wouldn't it seem odd for a spouse to insist on his or her own private line and then disappear into another room whenever the phone rang?

I understand the importance of privacy, but when it comes to husbands and wives, forging a lifetime of intimacy requires sacrifices. And personal privacy is one of them. Medical conditions, child-rearing issues, and important money matters should not be kept secret. And when it comes to whom you spend time with, and why, your life partner should have full access. That doesn't just apply to the partner who committed adultery, by the way. The electronic, phone, and web-based life of each spouse should be open to the other.

I recognize that in some situations that's not possible. If you work for the CIA, for example, you may need to have your own cell phone and e-mail (and no doubt a few extra passports under different aliases). There are similar considerations for bankers, doctors, pastors, and other professionals who have a duty to keep information confidential. But having your own line and your private e-mail address doesn't give you permission to have a private life.

Though, remember this: being transparent means giving complete access to your communications or connections. It doesn't mean that your spouse has access to all your thoughts. They're yours, they are inside of you, and it doesn't always help the relationship to share them censor-free. In the next chapter, we'll be talking about communicating feelings and thoughts. For now, remember that your spouse can't read your mind, but that your actions should be an open book.

Freedom of speech

With the right to see your partner's life comes great responsibility. You are free to look for evidence of affairs and to discuss concerns with your partner. But if you read each e-mail and then condemn, criticize, or disparage your mate because of the content sent by his or her (nonaffair) friends, you use that information as a weapon against your mate. If you do this, you will end up with an alienated spouse and will spur him or her on to finding some other way to communicate privately.

One couple I treated faced just this issue. This couple used the transparency policy because of Emily's concerns that Jason was having an affair. As far as anyone knows, Jason had never cheated on Emily, but this was one way of making sure that he didn't. Emily never did see any e-mails from paramours, but she was incensed that Jason would open up e-mails—sent by his old college buddies— that contained off-color jokes or soft porn photos. Emily was not concerned based on religious or moral grounds; it just seemed disrespectful to her. Jason argued (justifiably, I thought) that he couldn't be held responsible for what his friends sent him. He pointed out that he never forwarded the e-mails and never responded to them when they came.

At Emily's insistence, Jason had begun to ask his friends not to send any more lewd e-mails. In private, he told me that he felt embarrassed about having to sound so prudish to guys he used to play rugby with. As you might expect, his friends ignored his requests, still sent the crude jokes, until Emily pushed Jason to block them altogether.

In my opinion, Emily's approach abused the open-mail policy. She looked at all Jason's e-mails and held him responsible for their content, even if they had no direct impact on their relationship. If Emily had kept this up, she might have ultimately driven Jason to find an alternative hidden way to communicate with friends, thus opening up the door for an affair. When Emily realized that challenging Jason on his guy relationships was pushing him away, she stopped commenting on their e-mails. She still read them, and she still hated them, but that was her problem, not his, so she kept mum. Jason told me, "The marriage has been much happier since the change, but I still try to be very respectful about her feelings." In fact, he points out that since she has stopped harping on him, he's even more assertive about asking his friends to act respectfully when it comes to e-mails.

Open or vulnerable?

It is possible for anyone to have a see-through marriage, but it is not easy for some people. Many of my patients have trust issues. For them, being open means that they are exposing themselves to circumstances that could come back to hurt them. Sometimes this fear is just an inborn character trait. Sometimes it was taught from an early age by parents who were suspicious by nature. Some of my clients have been victims of abuse or incest during their childhoods and, for them, the ability to trust comes with great difficulty. For a person who is trust challenged, something as simple as keeping private one's own phone, or one's own Facebook entourage, acts to establish a sense of security.

Remember, your spouse is an individual who you promised to love forever, someone you walk in on in the bathroom, someone who has walked you to the door when you were too drunk to do it alone, someone you have had sex with, perhaps even who was there when you gave birth. In many interactions on many occasions your mate has gotten to know you intimately. In my opinion, being able to look at your e-mail, by comparison, is not that big a deal.

If you are reading this and feel very anxious about the possibility of your life partner having full access to your communications, this may reflect something about you or your partner that is worth taking a look at. If your partner misreads every e-mail or text, then (as I discussed in chapter 2) getting a psychiatric or psychological evaluation could help clarify the diagnosis of delusional disorder—jealous type, also known as "pathological jealousy." If your mate's behavior falls within normal range, then it may be time for you to make an appointment with a professional therapist to see whether your own trust issues are interfering with your ability to establish intimacy with your partner.

Friends parting ways

One posting to my message board illustrates the process of discovering an affair (or near affair), and how a couple works through the process of sharing the responsibility of ending inappropriate communication and reconnecting in the marriage.

My husband and I have been married for three years. We are in our mid-twenties. I entered into this marriage with trust issues; it was always something that caused me to snoop, etc. We spoke, and my husband assured me that I had no reason not to trust him and that I needed to let go of my fears. Fast forward six months, and I had made progress to the point that I was almost 100 percent trusting him. Last week, for whatever reason (divine intervention?), I looked into his phone. I found a text where he was breaking a friendship off with a friend who was a coworker. The first text was basically saying that they couldn't be friends because it is "a fine line between friendship and more." She argued but he stood pretty firm (she's def one of those kinda women).

A few weeks after that there is a text where she told him about her bad day at work and he says whatever about it and the conversation ends with him saying "nice talking to you. . ." Then, two weeks ago she sends a picture of herself and he says very nice and they chat about her birthday.

Of course I immediately bring the phone to him and ask for an explanation of the texts.

During our discussion he is extremely open and tells me they were work friends. She had invited him to lunch one day and things started from there. He said he basically cut it off with her via text because a few months before the actual text took place he distanced himself from her, because he knew the friendship was wrong and wanted it to stop. She texted and asked why he was so cold and that's how the "they couldn't be friends" text started. He said any texts that took place after the February "can't be friends" text were basically just trying to keep it cordial. Over the last seven days, he has been very open to discussion and will explain every last detail. He is firm in telling me it wasn't an emotional affair and he never turned to her for anything. It was just a friendship that he knew from the get go shouldn't have been.

The lies are what get me. He has been firm that nothing was worth lying for and he deeply regrets lying. I do believe that he is truly sorry. I feel like the only way I can move on is by accepting what happened and looking toward forgiveness, yet I'm finding it difficult to understand it all. Part of me wants to contact her, but he said he will contact her (visibly to me) and let her know to please leave him be. I feel resolution even after typing this, but I still feel hurt.

He did take steps to break it off with her and even verbalized that to her three months ago. They still exchanged texts, even two weeks ago. I know they weren't "bad," but (1) he was still in contact and (2) he did say "nice talking to you" and other "friendly" things. I feel like he wasn't cutting it off because of those texts. One of the exchanges took place around 10 p.m., so we were home together, and that certainly stings. He keeps assuring me that any text that took place after was just "cordial" (and, he admits, stupid still).

My professional opinion

This post illustrates how open communication can help couples work together to form good boundaries. It also highlights the concept of "slippery slope" of infidelity. Most people don't have affairs because they intend to; they "slip into" it through a series of increasingly less innocent interactions. But, if I had this woman in my office, here's what I would say:

1   Yes, he had interactions that you weren't aware of. At first, it didn't seem like something he *should* tell you about (a partner doesn't automatically tell another about every interaction with a person of the opposite sex).

2   Once he began to realize that the interactions were not so innocent, he then felt he *couldn't* tell you, because you'd react (understandably) with anger and perhaps fear. Your hubby isn't

alone in this dynamic—he's like many people who have done something wrong and want to avoid accountability. Ever hear the expression "what she doesn't know won't hurt her"? In that statement lies a truth; many people lie because they don't want their significant others to be hurt. Of course, they also lie to protect themselves. From what you tell me, I see no evidence that he is an evil man.

3 Once he saw the interaction start to move in the wrong direction, he took the steps to break it off. No, he didn't involve you (few marriages are strong enough to know how to share in these actions). But he took the initiative to make things right.

4 Once you "caught" him, he (apparently) was honest with you. That *is* unusual and is cause for some kudos on his part. You also deserve kudos for being able to approach him, rather than rip him to shreds. You asked him everything you wanted to know, and you got answers to your questions.

5 All in all, this was an aborted possible affair-in-the-making. In an ideal world, it never would have happened, but he did his level best to set things right.

6 Should you forgive? That's up to you. (In chapter 8 we will talk more about forgiveness.) In his mind, he withheld information because of fears that you would reject him if you found out. If you fail to forgive, withdraw your love, or punish him, then you end up reinforcing his beliefs. Something to think about. It sounds like this event may be a great opportunity for you to grow closer to each other.

One of the most important lessons of this story was that this couple's ability to recover from an affair depends in no small part on their willingness to open a dialogue about it.

❧ STEP 4: MAKE TIME TO TALK

At some point the person who has been cheated on has some questions that need to be answered. And at some point the cheating spouse has to answer them. As I noted earlier in the chapter, you probably haven't had a lot of experience navigating this issue, and, since this chapter is about what to do after an affair has ended, this step revolves around four essential guidelines, encompassing a policy that I've coined: "Do ask, do tell."

"Do ask, do tell" guidelines

1   The person who was cheated on may ask the person who cheated any question that he or she wishes about the events of the affair.

2   The person who cheated must answer all questions openly and completely.

3   The person who was cheated on may ask for any clarifications about the events of the affair he or she thinks reasonable.

4   The person who cheated must answer all questions openly and completely.

Your marriage has been through a lot and you've lived through it. Do you really have to talk about it? Sometimes couples are afraid that opening up a discussion is like pouring salt in the wound. Talking about it, they reason, will just make things worse. I take a firm and consistent approach on keeping an open dialogue because I have faith in the process of healing and the active role that each of you plays in it.

The person whose partner has strayed will usually only ask as much as he or she is ready to understand. Sometimes the questioning happens in stages; sometimes it happens all at once. If that person does not have a chance to have his or her questions answered, and instead imagines what happened, the visualizations that pass through the mind are often more frightening than the truth. Peggy Vaughan, founder of the internationally recognized Beyond Affairs Network, had surveyed thousands of infidelity survivors and written books and many scholarly articles. Far and away, the most helpful part of their recovery was the truthful revelation of the details according to the wishes of the inquiring spouse.

From the Web: We Can Handle Truth Better Than Lies

Always be truthful about questions of infidelity in the existing relationship. If it hurts you to tell your woman that you've been unfaithful, think of how *she's* going to feel if she ever finds out the truth about the guy she loves. Look, it's a selfless act that will let her move on if she cannot remain in the relationship, and she deserves to know who she's giving herself away to.

I'm coming from a personal perspective, because my man cheated on me, never told me about it, then his brother started dating the woman involved, and we all hung out together for a time, until the brother broke up with her and told me about it in a fit of rage. He told me what a fool I was for being with his brother. Of course, my husband denied it until one day (a year and half later) I was sitting at work and out of the blue it hit me. It was true. Call it ESP, or whatever, but after a series of arguments, he (and she) admitted it, and I was devastated. I tried forgiveness, and we even got married, believe it or not, but the question always remains, "Why did he do this to me?"

I've never cheated on him, but I don't feel the same anymore, at all. I question his capacity to love, and though he swears he always loved me, "it was just a mistake one night drinking," the fact remains that this is not the man I thought he was. And the future? Some days, I don't even want a future with him, in spite of all the forgiveness I can muster. It's ruined our love life. So for all of you who think you can do this "just once" and it won't matter, try this instead: tell your wife you want to go out and play around, and give her the right to find someone she can trust. We can handle truth far better than lies.

—Darlene, 34, one year into her second marriage

It's the trust, stupid!

Recovering from infidelity, stripped to its essentials, is all about rebuilding trust. Once the person who had an affair has broken vows, the other partner will always be left to wonder if that person can ever be trusted again. When the faithful partner seeks out information about an affair, he or she believes that knowing is a vital part of recovering. Sharing in an open dialogue allows information to flow in a way that fills in the gaps. When the cheated poses questions to the cheater, the cheater will have a choice, "Do I tell everything?" or "Do I decide what I do and don't tell based on my own estimation of what's best for me and my partner?" Which do you think is more likely to build trust?

While I was writing this book, I presented a seminar on infidelity at the annual conference of the American Psychiatric Association. As I transitioned from the "what is infidelity" hour into the "what to do about it" hour, I presented my four "Time to Talk" rules. Incredibly (to me) many of the psychiatrists in the audience objected. Their main concern is that the person who had an affair may irrevocably damage the marriage by revealing something so offensive that it will precipitously drive away his or her partner. Some (not all) felt that it was up to the unfaithful partner to decide what to tell, and he or she should trust his or her judgment about what the other spouse is able to hear. *Yeah*, I thought, as I politely listened to these learned practitioners of my profession, *because the unfaithful one was able to demonstrate such good judgment before!* My peers' opinions notwithstanding, I believe the only way to reestablish trust and begin to forgive is to stop withholding, stop lying, stop finessing the answer, and be truthful. Except when it's dangerous . . .

Exceptions to the guidelines

Not every case of withholding the truth is a sign of poor judgment. There are some situations where withholding the whole truth is prudent. I treated one couple, Luigi and Maureen, who were in their mid-thirties and had four school-aged children at home. Luigi was so distraught about a suspected affair between Maureen and her coworker that he tried to kill himself. His wife admitted to an emotional—but not sexual—affair and promised never to see the man again. During a brief interaction with Maureen, I learned that Luigi had a history of uncontrolled violence at home and that "if he ever found out that I actually did sleep with the man, he would kill me."

Obviously, Maureen is in a dangerous marriage, and I worry about whether she should be with Luigi at all. But Maureen insists that in all other regards she values and treasures the marriage and points out that Luigi has never actually caused her any serious physical harm. There are many such marriages. Adults can choose to be (or not to be) with powder keg spouses, but it's certainly understandable why Maureen would choose to protect herself by withholding information. In cases like hers, deviation from the four basic rules makes sense.

A situation like Maureen and Luigi's is the exception. You may be tempted to see yourself in it, though. You may be inclined to withhold the truth because "my spouse would be furious," or "my spouse would go into a deep depression," or "my spouse would totally withdraw from me." Anger or hurt feelings are not on the same level as murder; anger and hurt feelings have to be expected and tolerated. They are a natural consequence of the cheater's behavior. I understand that unraveling the details of an affair may cause you and your mate extreme pain, but I do not see this kind of pain as reasons for withholding the truth. In these cases you've done the crime, now you've got to do the time.

Sometimes the non-cheating partner has no questions. One client of mine is sure that her husband has had an affair because of some correspondence she uncovered. She has accused him; he has not denied it, but he hasn't admitted to it either. My client is angry and upset, but she won't ask him any more questions. "I know that if I hear the details, then I will not be able to stay in the marriage and protect my own sense of dignity. But I've invested twenty-five years in this relationship, so it's easier for me to be in ignorance and to move on with our lives." As I discuss in chapter 10, marriages stay together for many reasons despite affairs. In this case, the partner who has not cheated chooses to reduce her sense of pain by not asking and by simultaneously shutting out disturbing images in her mind.

Kind of sort of true

Obfuscation is part of the flame addiction. It's based on the mistaken belief that others will find you less reprehensible if you can just keep them from knowing about how badly you have let them down. Cheaters typically find every rationalization to withhold the truth from a partner. If you and your partner are reading this book because an affair has been uncovered, then you already know that efforts to keep secrets from your partner have not worked in the past. I can tell you that they are not likely to work in the future, either.

Here's a typical dialogue to illustrate the problem of failure of full disclosure:

> She: How many times did you see her?
>
> He: I don't really remember.
>
> She: I don't want an exact number. Five? Fifty? How many times would you guess?
>
> He: I honestly don't know. Maybe five. Maybe fifteen. I've already apologized, why do we have to keep talking about it?

In this case, the person cheating withholds information from the person cheated on. There's a big difference between five and fifteen. Does her husband, who can recall the batting average of every player on his fantasy baseball team, really not know how often he had seen his mistress? Neither partner is going to be happy with this flow of dialogue, yet I hear conversations like this all the time. She thinks that if she asks often enough, he'll eventually tell. He would be happier if she would just stop asking. If he puts up enough roadblocks, he reasons, she'll just forget about it and never bring it up again. Not likely.

She is getting increasingly frustrated. Being pushed away just piques her curiosity and worries even more. Left in the dark, she fears her worst nightmare is true. She begins to ask more and more often. He gets increasingly agitated at her badgering. Now, rather than talk about the affair, they begin to argue about her "nagging" and his withholding.

A truthful dialogue

Now let's look at a conversation using the rules:

She: How many times did you see her?

He: I saw her about six times, from February to May.

She: Where did you see her?

He: Usually we went to her apartment. She has a kid who would stay with her ex-husband for the weekends. I'd go over when I told you I was running to Home Depot.

She: Did you ever use our house?

He: No.

She: Did you ever think of me during all those times?

Can you see how, once the details are laid out, she can move from the where and when to the emotional effects of the affair? This isn't to say that each grain of information may not irritate, anger, or sadden her. But she asked, and he tells. And that process, regardless of the horrifying answers, is necessary to healing.

You'll note that I stopped the dialogue just as she was asking about his feelings and thoughts. Giving honest answers about the emotional impact of an affair is more complicated than answering who, where, and when. I recommend putting these discussions on hold until you read chapter the next chapter.

She: Did you ever think of me during all those times?

He: Yes, but I really don't know how to talk about that at this point. Is it okay if we read the next chapter and learn how to have these kinds of discussions before I answer you?

She: Okay, that's fair. I appreciate your telling me the details, though. I had thought it was only once that you met, so now I have to process my own feelings about this.

So far he and she are staying pretty unruffled. But, in real life, people aren't always able to stay to calm, cool, and collected. You may be worried that the conversation can get out of control. Consider this conversation:

She: Did you enjoy having sex with her?

He: Yes.

She: Did you like it better than sex with me?

He: That's complicated; I'd like to wait until we read the next chapter before I answer that.

She: I can see that that has to do with emotions, not facts. So I'll wait to talk to you about that. Did you have oral sex?

He: Yes, we had oral sex.

She: You on her or her on you?

He: Both.

She: That's disgusting! I can't believe you would do that to me! I don't want to hear any more!

This cannot be an easy conversation. She wants to know about the emotional impact of the affair but agrees to stick to tangible details. Nonetheless, she is extremely upset with how he answered. This dialogue illustrates how really tough questions can be asked. In this case, the person cheated on felt it was important to know about the kind of sex her husband had with the other woman. Even though she's disgusted, it is something she needed to know. In my experience, if the cheated partners don't want to know these details, they don't ask the questions. They set up their own filter; somehow their unconscious knows how much they are willing to hear. They either don't ask, or, as in the example above, they will stop listening when the details become too graphic or too overwhelming.

Asking nitty-gritty questions, however (as in the example above), is bound to increase the risk of getting nitty-gritty answers. People naturally try to avoid unpleasant experiences, so it's tempting to shy away from telling the noxious truth. But if the questions are asked, answering them is essential to rebuilding trust.

When does it end?

Above all, the unfaithful spouse worries that every truthful answer to a question will just raise more questions and that he or she will never be able to satisfy his or her partner. As one of my patients said, "She wants to examine every detail with a fine-toothed comb. I feel like it's an interrogation."

This is understandable. Like your favorite *Law and Order* episode, where the job of the cop is to break down the perpetrator and piece together the crime, the faithful partner sees the other as a criminal. Only when all the truth is uncovered can that partner see the whole picture. Only then can he or she decide what to do next.

In theory, anyway.

From a practical point of view, sometimes one partner has heard all the information the other has to share, yet he or she still feels like the whole truth remains hidden. That is because either the cheater is still hiding things or the person cheated on just can't be satisfied, even with 100 percent responsiveness to all the questions. It is maddening to the unfaithful spouse, who feels confused by the partner's refusal to accept his or her version of the truth. When exposed to a barrage of "I don't believe anything you say no matter what," the unfaithful spouse is at risk of withdrawing and giving up on the possibility of the marriage's ever moving forward.

If the cheated feels that there are still open questions, then most marriages stall out right here. The bottom line: at a certain point, the cheated just has to accept that the cheater has told everything there is to tell. It's not easy, because it involves trusting someone who has lied to you.

When couples have succeeded at doing the necessary tasks of unveiling, ending the other relationship, breaking off communication, and talking to each other about the events of the affair, the next challenge is to help each other explore the thoughts and feelings that occur during the affair. That's a different kind of talk altogether, and we'll address that in the next chapter.

7

Getting to the Heart of the Matter

My husband and I own a home and have three young children. I recently saw a video in his phone of him having sex with a woman. I confronted him about it and asked when it happened. He said it happened more than two years ago, at a time when I told him I didn't want to be married to him and I had kicked him out of our home. He said he thought our marriage was over, and he was angry, so he contacted an old female friend. They drank at a bar, and then she returned to the hotel where he said he stayed. He claimed he knew what he did was wrong and apologized. He said he never thought I would find out and didn't want to tell me because we got back together three or four days after I put him out.

I struggle with the fact that he recorded it on a cell phone and kept it. Further, he had unprotected sex. I feel so betrayed and don't know if I could forgive him. Am I wrong? Isn't it cheating, since we were legally married?

I am in such emotional turmoil. I can't sleep at night because I keep thinking about my husband being with another person. He told me that it is so difficult for him to talk about because he just wanted to forget it ever happened. I then asked when was the last time he spoke to her, and I asked him to be honest. He said he calls about once a month to see how she's doing, because her mother passed away. The only way he could have known would be if he had kept in touch after being intimate with her.

I have been crying so hard from my soul because I feel he has no remorse or regret, because if he did he would not have remained in contact with her. The idea that he kept in touch hurts more than the act of cheating that (he claimed) happened two years ago. Is this crazy for me to think? I also asked him to call the woman in front of me and tell her that I know and that they are no longer to be in contact, which he did. But I still do not feel any better.

I have never experienced such a deep pain caused from betrayal. In fact every time his phone rings or he gets a text message my heart races and I feel sick to my stomach. I don't know what to do.

Sean (another participant on the message board) responds:

There's no way not to feel torn apart by this. Let me offer you my experience as perhaps a way to help shed some light on the male perspective.

I cheated on my wife more than a decade ago. I was incredibly naive, and we both let our relationship drift into dangerous waters. We'd been together many years and then brought a child into our family. To make a long story short, I was unseated emotionally and intimately by my beloved baby. My very male reaction was to yearn desperately for my lost intimacy, and I found it online, which consummated in a weekend with another woman. Again, I was incredibly foolish/ignorant as to the devastation it would cause my marriage. I still did and do very much love my wife.

Stupidly, after it happened I wrote a detailed account of the weekend on my smart phone, which my wife discovered a month later. Very similar to your experience. I've wished to have that time back to do over again so many times, for I lost my wife's trust (really forever) and my own sense of integrity.

The question remains for us—for you two—where do you go from here? Do you have the elements of love and friendship that are worth

working on to salvage your marriage? Are there other compelling reasons
to stay together (children, a stable home)? From my experience, we made
it work for our children and our stable home. I'm not going to sugarcoat
this: our marriage has a gaping hole in it to this day where once stood *trust*,
honesty, and *intimacy*. On top of that there are the issues that led us to that
point—the children are still number one for her and now this is *my problem*
not hers.

I certainly take the blame for my decision to stray and can only accept
what forgiveness she has given me (I'm still in the house), but some of
the pain seems to be irreparable. That is my lasting consequence. I was
very sorry and remorseful. I'm not sure your husband is, or maybe he's still
processing it. I immediately let go of the other woman; that *has* to happen
to have any hope for healing. If your husband loves you, even if he isn't
feeling it now, he is in for a lifetime of remorse and pain for his mistake. I can
vouch for that!

Never take your love for granted, and by that same token, *Love* can heal if
two are willing.

Emma's and Sean's stories walk us through the phases of infidelity
from the discovery, to the unveiling, to the termination of an affair.
In Emma's story, we even see the all-too-often example, as I describe
in chapter 6, of an unfaithful spouse holding onto a relationship even
when the affair has ended. In both of these cases, the husband con-
fesses to the affair, ends the sex, acknowledges his wrongdoing, and
seeks reconciliation with his mate. In just about every way, these stories illustrate the process of going through Step 1 through Step 4 that
I described in the previous chapter.

But these two vignettes reveal to us much more than the "how to"
of managing the post-affair fallout. They also point out the powerful emotional impact of an affair on the marriage and how difficult
rebuilding can be. When Emma's husband and Sean recommit to the
marriage, they face a relationship much different from the one they
strayed from. Their wives are emotionally scarred from the husbands'
behavior. Something must happen to allow the marriage to heal.

What is needed for a couple to push aside the devastation of the affair? This is where Step 5 starts: it's time to talk about what's going on inside.

❧ TALK

What's the truth?

The previous chapter reviewed the very specific steps needed to begin the process of having a conversation about the affair. Do you remember when the wife asked if the husband preferred sex with the other person to sex with her? The husband replied, "That's complicated; I'd like to wait until we read the next chapter before I answer that."

Several times in the previous chapter, when I counseled you to talk about what happened during the affair, I advised you to put off talking about its emotional impact until you were ready. Too many people try to dig deep into this level of conversation before they know how. If you've worked through the last chapter, then you've started the work of unpeeling the onion. Now it's time to work on how to talk about the emotions of the affair.

Most marriage counselors are dogmatic; they insist that each partner in the marriage be completely honest with each other at all times. But common sense and basic decency make this a very difficult proposition. Take my friend Claude. During his honeymoon in Bora Bora, Claude and his wife were relaxing in the white sands of a perfect beach when he noticed a woman in a bikini standing on the edge of the dock. He casually mentioned to his wife how stunning that woman standing there was. His wife was aghast. There he was, married to her for a mere two days, and already he was noticing (and commenting on!) other women. Moreover, his wife told him, if he thought this stranger on the beach was spectacular, what must he think of his new bride?

I tell you this story neither to defend my friend nor to point out how dopey he is. Rather, it's a cautionary tale. By sharing the "truth" with his wife, he left her with a very bad feeling about herself and about him. Such honesty did nothing to improve the honeymoon, although I suppose it was helpful in that it taught him a lesson about marriage: it's not a good idea to share every thought or every observation that enters your mind.

What you think and what you say

Let's start with a simple example outside of the highly charged subject of marriage. Suppose you sit on the sidelines as you watch your daughter play striker for her soccer team. There are seconds left in the game, and a ball flies across the opponent's goal just at the level where she could head it in for a goal. Instead, she takes a step back to try to trap it with her feet, and a defensive player kicks it out of bounds to secure a victory for the other team.

You approach your daughter after the game, as she shakes her head in self-disgust. You wish to be honest with her and may choose from the following statements:

- "Your poor decision probably lost the game for your team."
- "Your friends may all be mad at you."
- "You lacked skill on the ball field."
- "You made a good effort and will be sure to learn from this."

All of these comments are true. But good parenting dictates that you don't say everything that comes into your mind. We learn as parent, coworker, child, and friend that filtering truthful input can help improve relationships and avoid causing other people hurt. That's why most parents would choose the last option.

I use the example of the soccer match not only to demonstrate how saying good things builds strong egos but also to remind you that for any one situation there are many truths. When discussing soccer, you can build up one truth and put another out of you mind. When it comes to having an honest discussion with your mate about your affair, you have to choose which truth you share with him or her.

This does not mean that I recommend you lie. Instead, you must be thoughtful about the impact of your statements.

A soft touch

There's another reason to tread lightly when sharing the truth. Couples who have very secure marriages may be willing to give their partners the benefit of the doubt when confronted with a painful truth. But when couples are healing from infidelity, the marriage often isn't strong enough to withstand brutal honesty. The person on the receiving end of the information may easily feel hurt by truthful comments. He or she may misinterpret information and be prone to view it in the most negative light.

Going back to the hypothetical couple above: When she asks him: "Did you like sex with her better than sex with me?" one honest answer is: "Yes. It was awesome and much more exciting than sex with you." That might reasonably reflect the truth of anyone having an affair, since (as we discussed in chapter 4) the surges in brain dopamine involved in having any novel stimuli, particularly an affair, heighten physiologic arousal and are very pleasurable.

Another honest answer is: "You and I don't have enough sex for me to know!" This is meant to deflect attention away from his transgressions and label her as the cause of the affair. It borders on the truth, because they may be having less sex than they had been in the past. In that regard, they would be among the vast majority of Americans, whose rate of sexual activity declines after marriage and children.

Another truthful answer is: "No. Being with a new sexual partner was exciting, but the amount of shame I felt over what I had done made the experience feel worse, not better. Sex is much more meaningful with you, and I value it above all."

Three truths, and one important moment in your marriage. Often, a straight-from-the-hip answer is selected out of a grab bag of honest answers, and the one you choose may be tinged with something other than the best of intentions. You may wish to brag, wound, get even, or justify. You can find a true statement that will accomplish any of these conscious or unconscious goals. If you wish to recover from the marriage, you must be thoughtful before you answer questions about your feelings.

❧ TO THE ONE WHO HAD THE AFFAIR

Think before you speak

If you have committed infidelity, here are some principles to keep in mind as you begin to talk with your partner truthfully about your feelings:

- Take a good self-inventory.
- Consider your spouse's feelings before you talk.
- Don't couch things in a criticism, overt or hidden, of your mate.
- Don't use a confession as a means for you to feel better if it means hurting your spouse.

Take a good self-inventory

Before you can talk with your mate about what caused the affair and how you felt about it before, during, and after, you have to stand up to the mirror and do a considerable amount of self-exploration. When you try to answer a question about why you do the things you do, you must distinguish between reason and rationalization. Before talking about the affair, let's look at an example of a "small crime": stealing a piece of penny candy from an open bin at a store. The *reason* you stole it may be lack of morals, inability to suppress your urges, or a belief that you wouldn't get caught—not very attractive attributes, but, then, stealing isn't a very attractive act. *Rationalization*, in contrast, would explain your lifting the candy like this: "They wouldn't have left it out unless they expected people to steal it," "No one will know the difference if I take one candy," or "I was hungry—what else was I supposed to do?"

To figure out your reasons (not your rationalizations), go back and look at chapters 4 and 5, where I discuss physical and emotional needs. We can muse about why Tiger Woods has dalliances, but you need to identify what needs you tried to satisfy with *your* affair. For most people, there will be more than one need. Most needs are internal (for example, the need to be loved) and some are external (for example, the need for orgasm). If you stick to the simplest external explanations, such as saying to your partner, "You were just ignoring me too much, and I couldn't take being put down anymore," then your spouse is left with the message "It's not me, it's you." That's not right.

Here are some reasons (and in some cases rationalizations) why people have affairs (there are some crossovers with the list in chapter 5). Look at the list, and then look at yourself in the mirror. If you can't be honest with yourself about why you strayed, how are you going to be honest with your mate?

Sexual enjoyment
Curiosity
Excitement
Intellectual sharing
Understanding
Companionship
Ego-bolstering
Career advancement
Getting even with spouse

As you look at the list, do you see clues about what may have contributed to your infidelity? Are there reasons you have thought of that don't appear on this list? In some cases it may just not be possible to make sense out of why you did what you did. But don't pass the affair off glibly as "a one-time mistake." Find professional help, if needed: sit down with an unbiased counselor who can help you figure out what propelled you in the direction of an affair.

From the Web: The Worst Thing

My wife and I dated, off and on, for thirteen years before we married in 2007. This past summer I had an affair with a coworker, and my wife found out. There were, so I thought, several variables that played a part in me drifting away from our relationship. I have since come to terms with the fact that no matter what was going on in our lives, going outside of our marriage was the worst thing that I could have done to us. The months since my affair have consisted of both high and low points. Long story short, I hurt my wife in a way that I never thought possible and I am trying to do all that I can to reassure her that she is my home and it is with her that I want/need to be. I love her more than I could ever express with words. I wish to let her know that I will *never* hurt her this way again.

Consider your spouse's feelings before you talk

Do you and your spouse feel differently about how often to go shopping? Do you feel differently about whether playing Monopoly is fun? Do you feel differently about whether you'd consider running a bed and breakfast? Your life partner and you have different feelings about many things, so don't expect your mate to feel the same way about your style of communication as you do. For instance, some people crack a joke to relieve tension, but their mates feel that humor during stressful times minimizes the gravity of the situation. Some partners may feel that the only place to have a discussion is in public, like a restaurant, but the other may freeze up with social anxiety. Still other people feel the best way to work things through is to write long letters describing all dimensions of emotions, but their partner may feel that reading and responding to such letters is burdensome. Your partner didn't ask for you to have this affair, and, now that he or she is asking for a serious talk about it, you should consider how he or she best receives information before you decide how to address things.

One of the keys to happy marriages (we'll talk more about this in chapter 11) is to get to know your partner's communication style. This involves not only understanding what she or he says, but also what goes unspoken. Reading your partner involves long periods of observation, occasional direct inquiry, and even testing out your hypotheses, for example, saying, "When you raise your voice, I think you are angry. Am I reading you right?" When you have a discussion with your partner, consider how he or she would like to be addressed and what kinds of words work best. Does he respond to action words, such as "I think," or to emotional words, like "I feel"? Are long explanations helpful to her, or do short statements better hit the mark? If he or she doesn't respond the way you expect, maybe it has to do with your presentation, and not with your partner's attitude.

Don't couch things in a criticism, overt or hidden, of your mate

As you try to make sense of your transgressions during the time you were having an affair, it's easy to point the finger of blame in the direction of your partner. A firestorm of controversy hit the TV airwaves in 2010 when Oprah Winfrey asked Gary Neuman, the author of a book called *The Truth about Cheating*, to explain his findings. He stated that many of the one hundred unfaithful men he interviewed for his book said that the main cause of the affair was a lack of emotional and sexual responsiveness from their wives. The hullabaloo arose because it appeared that these men, and the man who wrote the book about them, were saying that wives' behavior caused the affair. In its review of the book, *Publisher's Weekly* wrote that Neuman challenges "women to revise assumptions about marriage, make immediate behavioral changes and forge new bonds with their husbands, thereby deterring future dalliances. While some wives might find this book helpful, it is perhaps more likely that readers will wish that the author had devoted more time to holding the cheating husband responsible for his actions rather than putting the onus on wives to take preventive—and dubiously effective—measures."

Whether the wife bears some responsibility isn't the issue. Everyone's relationship could use a little work, and all mates could and should work harder to forge stronger bonds with their partners.

But when someone whose life is turned upside down is told that he or she is responsible for their trauma—no, it just doesn't fly.

Even if you feel your relationship problems contributed to your unhappiness (and in many cases they have), you should still be very clear that the decision to have an affair was yours to make. You cannot blame your partner. When it comes to discussing your feelings and thoughts with your mate, the word "I" should be front and center, and the word "you" barely spoken.

Don't make yourself feel better if it means hurting your spouse

Affairs are rotten things. If you've had an affair, you probably feel remorse for what you have done. Talking about the affair will give you an opportunity to discuss its emotional impact on you: the confusion, the ambivalence, the shame, and, perhaps, your passion to make amends. Sometimes baring your soul may feel like redemption for you, but it may be torture for your partner. Be considerate of how your words are affecting your mate. If, early on in the process of disclosure, you pour out your heart looking for sympathy or forgiveness, your partner may start feeling pretty annoyed. In the context of the pain he or she is experiencing, the idea that your torment must be given full attention just doesn't seem fair.

You may feel tormented. You've done a bad thing. But restrain yourself from trying to draw the attention away from your mate's experience. Instead, pace your own disclosure of emotional pain so it doesn't exceed your partner's.

TO THE PERSON WHO HAS BEEN CHEATED ON

Can you handle the truth?

When I've talked about disclosure with my patients, the person whose spouse had an affair often asks me, "How can you ask my cheating spouse to withhold anything? Shouldn't I be able to hear the absolute truth?" Let me reiterate: when it comes to the "what happened" events of the infidelity, your spouse must tell all. But I want you to appreciate that emotional truths are a lot more complicated and that thoughtful answers can foster some very meaningful discussions.

In the 1992 film *A Few Good Men*, Jack Nicholson plays a navy colonel who gradually loses his patience because a military lawyer, played by Tom Cruise, incessantly needles him. After bobbing and weaving, and doing everything in his ability to avoid giving details on the death of a sailor, Nicholson finally succumbs to the irritating lawyer and shouts his now famous line, "You can't handle the truth!"

The experience of being betrayed by your mate is traumatic. It leaves you with doubts about yourself and doubts about the entire story of your marriage. You will carry on many self-dialogues as you play and replay scenes from your marriage and try to make sense out of every minute, every interaction. At each interval, you will be seeking information from your mate, the very one who caused you all this pain. As your spouse works with you to fill in the gaps, I ask, what are you going to do with this information?

Discussing marital transgressions sometimes feels like a courtroom drama. You put all the evidence out for your spouse to see. He or she has a clear-cut duty to deliver honest responses. But let me ask you: Can you handle the truth? Will you believe it? Will you shout "You're lying!" to every possible response? Will you break down in tears or turn stone cold? Will you throw coals on a burning rage? Will you simply drift away mentally, shut down, and go through the motions while inwardly feeling nothing? You have an opportunity to do some relationship building here, but it will take foresight and patience.

Listen to things you don't want to hear

You can steer the course of your marriage with how you handle the truth that your husband or wife tells. If you have been the victim of infidelity, you may feel that you've been through enough and that your partner should do all the work from here on. But you absolutely need good skills of your own to help you get through this. Here are a few important concepts to remember when you ask your partner about the emotional aspects of the affair:

- Take your own self-inventory.
- Don't be a mind detective.
- Listen without judgment.
- Let your partner know when and what you're ready to hear.
- Be a conduit, not a roadblock, for conversation.

Take your own self-inventory

What are you upset about in the affair? How do you balance all the intense emotions inside of you? The upcoming dialogues with your partner are bound to be emotionally charged. First, try to sort through your own feelings. I recommend taking this step because, if things aren't sorted out in your own head, then you'll lose your bearings when you and your mate discuss the affair. When he or she looks at you and says: "What do you want from me?" you'll actually have an answer based on careful analysis, not simply a snappy answer to a stupid question. Moreover, it will help you structure the conversation in a way that will help you meet your goals.

You undoubtedly are flooded with different feelings about the affair and the impact it has had on you and your marriage. Here are some of the emotions described by people who have contributed to my website:

Serina: I get suspicious and insecure . . . then I make myself miserable with "checking" on him, getting internally angry, mulling over the past.

Elena: I am very unhappy. I would rather die than face the shame of a divorce. I am very sad that I have disappointed the Lord.

Sheila: I felt great pain and there's no solution for that.

Nicole: I have been dealing with this for so long that I am actually past the point of crying. He killed a part of me that will never come back. This changed me into a hateful, angry, sad, pessimistic person.

Adam: This is painful but I don't know how to talk to her about it. I don't know where to start other than to try to be the best husband I can.

Abby: Things will never be the same. My heart is broken, and I feel as if I'll never be able to trust him again.

Kora: I am the wife who looked the other way, because I am afraid of being abandoned again.

Matt: Am I over it? Heck no, but I'm not wallowing in my own despair, depression, and grief.

Cindy: I have never felt such hurt, shame, humiliation, and betrayal in all my life. The pain is just so unbearable.

Richard: I can't get over the thoughts of her with someone else.

Now think of your emotional response. Start by writing a list of all the feelings that have been stirred up by the affair. Every adjective that comes to mind. The table on the next page will help you begin the process of delving into your emotions. In the first column, write all of the feelings you can think of.

In the next column, rate the intensity of the feeling from one to ten, with one being very faint, hardly noticeable, and ten representing the most intensity you could possibly imagine. Of course, the strength of the emotions will vary from day to day, so for this exercise, just rate how you feel *right now,* or how you felt during the previous day.

In the third column, next to each emotion, I'd like you to take the opportunity to take stock of the trigger of the emotion. You may place a check next to any (or all) of the three options: you, the affair, or your mate. If you list "sad," for example, you might indicate that it is *the affair* that makes you sad. If you write "hate," you might indicate that this is directed toward your *partner.* For "anger," some people would endorse that they feel angry with their *partner,* others at the

Feeling	Intensity (1–10)	Direction			What will make it better from . . .		
		Me	Affair	Spouse	Me	Him	Me

Self-assessment of feelings after an affair

fact that the *affair* took place, still another might say the anger is with *myself*. In the examples above, Kora writes that she was afraid of being abandoned. That would be an example of an emotion whose source is herself, so Kora would check off "me" in this section.

The last two columns focus on what it will take for negative emotions to go away. (These are feelings that you would like to go away, so if you have included positive emotions such as "relief" or "clarity" in your first column, then you will not feel any desire to turn those around.) In the second to last column, write what you think *your partner can do* that will help a negative feeling get better. In the last column, write what *you can do* to reduce or eliminate the negative feeling. What you come up with in these last two columns may or may not be practical solutions, but it doesn't really matter. This is an opportunity to be creative about how you and your partner can move past these intense negative emotions. On the next page is an example of how Erica, a 28-year-old woman in her fourth year of marriage, filled out the chart.

As you work on this chart, you will start to make some very important observations. Before doing this exercise, you may have felt flooded with all the emotions you have been dealing with and confused by some of them. By sorting through these feelings one at a time, you will begin to get a clearer picture of the sensations going through your head. You will also recognize that you don't feel all the emotions with the same force; on some days, some will predominate; on other days, different ones will prey on your mind. You'll also appreciate that not all of your feelings are the direct product of your spouse's behavior; some come about from your own "baggage." That's important to keep in mind, because, as you sort through what you need from your partner to heal, you'll also need to keep in mind what you need from *you*.

Don't be a mind detective

You needed to be a detective when it came to the who, what, and where of an affair but excavating for facts is less complex than digging for feelings. One of the most common complaints I hear from

Feeling	Intensity (1–10)	Direction			What will make it better from …	
		Me	Affair	Spouse	Him	Me
Sad	8		x	x	Reassure me that it won't happen again and that he loves me	Try to move on and learn from the experience
Angry	5		x	x	Let me vent my angry feelings	Vent my feeling to James and close friends
Sick to my stomach	10		x		Nothing. Only time can cure that	Try to put detail of the affair out of my head and focus on other things
Guilty	5	x			Show appreciation for the thing I do for him	Understand that it was not my fault

Sample of a completed self-assessment

people who begin talking about infidelity is that their partner, usually the one cheated on, tries to interpret the emotions of the other partner. I know why you would do that: you are probably trying to explain why your spouse would do something so awful, and, lacking any good explanation on his or her part, you are trying to figure it out yourself. I understand; but if I could just say one word on the subject—stop!

Not being honest about *what* happened—a necessity for the unfaithful partner—is different from not being honest about *why* it happened. Your mate's inability to answer probing questions into why he or she had an affair and to tell you how he or she feels about it do not prove your spouse is hiding anything from you. Instead your partner might be hiding things from himself or herself. He or she might forever be unable to make sense of the actions leading to the affair. The fact is you don't know why your spouse claims ignorance. When you try to figure out what your spouse's behavior denotes by psychoanalyzing your partner or trying to read your partner's mind, not only do you run the risk of being dead wrong, but you also risk really ticking off your spouse.

Another example of detective work is when the affected partner seeks contradictions in what the cheating partner describes. Examples include "How can you tell me that you didn't care about her when you chose to buy her flowers?" or "You tell me I'm a priority, but when I needed your help with the yard work, you're meeting him for coffee!" Pointing out your partner's inconsistencies in the "who, what, and where" takes place as a natural way on your part to put the pieces together. But try doing it as part of a discussion of thoughts and emotions, and you will come off like a spousal CSI, stirring resentment, irritation, and eventually withdrawal.

Ultimately, positive discussion should work toward both partners having a better understanding of the events preceding, during, and following the affair. In a collaborative way, you can both do some mental sleuthing. But if it's done as a "Gotcha!" approach, particularly when you are trying to prove what your partner feels, no one wins.

Listen without judgment

One of the reasons I ask you to take your own emotional pulse early on in this process is because you will have very strong gut reactions as your partner's description of the affair unfolds. You are not made of stone; of course your mate's words will stir up passionate reactions on your part. However strong your urge to rise up, strike out, protest, storm out, or lament, the best advice I can give you is to keep mum during these heart-to-heart discussions. You've asked your mate to open up his or her heart. You may hear some earth-shattering revelation or you may hear USDA prime BS, but whatever your partner begins to discuss, you should allow the free flow of discussion without shutting it down.

When I recommend this to people, they object on the grounds that subjecting themselves to be passive listeners is like being revictimized. Yes, you have been the victim, but in the vast majority of cases, your pain is the *by-product* of your mate's behavior, not the primary *goal*. (Occasionally, but rarely, people will say that they had an affair in order to wound their partner in some way.) The fact that you were hurt will need to be addressed, but if you jump in too soon with your side of the story, it will give a message to your spouse that you don't want to hear his or hers. There is always a risk that the more your partner talks, the more he or she will begin to believe his set of rationalizations and lies. In most cases, though, once your mate has begun the process of dissecting emotions, everyone begins to get a clearer picture of what was going on. Your ability to listen helps facilitate bonding between the both of you.

From the Web: The Hardest Thing You'll Ever Do

As soon as you suspect an affair, that is the time for open dialogue and communication. I sat through a year of my husband's "friendship" with a gal from work. He wasn't willing to give up this friendship for an entire year. However, I *knew* my husband and what was taking place was quite out of character for him. Because of this, I truly felt it was worth it to wait this out.

Meanwhile, I didn't just sit there like a doormat hoping he would come around. I didn't sit there demanding that he stop seeing her (okay . . . that did happen two or three times. . .).

What I *did* was *listen* to my husband, all the while knowing he really "liked" her and wasn't willing to give her up and was still sharing things with her on a daily basis. It wasn't easy. He told me the hurts he had been carrying, caused by me. He told me how unappreciated he felt. He told me a lot.

It hurt like hell to hear those things, because on top of *that* hurt was the hurt I was feeling because of what he was doing. I listened anyway. And I changed. I became the person he married and that I was too stubborn to be as the years went by. It wasn't even that hard because I *knew* what was at stake: the love of my life.

I can honestly say, in listening to my husband and making the changes I needed to make, I am a hundred times the person I was before all this took place. And the changes I made have been internalized. I don't even think anymore about whether to apologize or not, it is just a part of my being. Same goes for so many things.

Be willing to listen without being defensive. The hardest thing you'll ever do, but so worth it.

Let your partner know when and what you need to hear

Going through an affair is hard work, and it's work you've probably never had to reckon with before. So there may be things that you need from your conversations and you find yourself getting frustrated because you're not hearing them. Many couples resolve this problem with one simple act: they ask for what they want.

Latoyan had been married for only two years when she had consulted me about her husband's affair. "I'm so frustrated because all I want to know is that he still loves me. But he's so busy making excuses for why the affair happened that I never get what I want out of our discussions." I suggested that she tell her husband what she needs and help him help her feel satisfied. I told Latoyan how open-ended discussions get the ball rolling, but sometimes you need to narrow the focus. I also explained that she may need to be very specific and help walk her husband through the steps of getting what she wants.

Many partners (usually husbands) are reluctant to say what their partner wants them to say. Here's the rationale that someone like Latoyan's husband might cite: "I do love her. I love her very much. But I'm afraid if I say it because she is asking me to say it, that she won't believe it." If I were counseling them together I would tell the husband to stop overthinking the situation and give Latoyan what she needs. But since I have only Latoyan in the office (and since I have you reading this section of the book), I can help her coach her partner into getting what she wants.

First, be very direct. Instead of saying, "It would be nice to hear some kind words," say, "I need you to say you love me." If that doesn't work, say, "Say 'I love you.'"

Second, be willing to coach your partner through what you need, and, if possible, use humor. In Latoyan's case, I told her to grab her husband's cheeks and lips and help him form the words.

Third, give lots of positive feedback, even when it's a close call. When Latoyan's husband said, "You know I love you," she was tempted to scream, "That's not what I wanted! I want to hear the words!" Instead she said, "It's nice to hear you acknowledge your love for me. That means a lot. " Later, she can help him give her more of what she needs by reiterating, "I know you love me, but I need to hear the words, 'I love you,' from your mouth."

For Latoyan, she needed words of love. You may need the same, or you may need other things. If you go back to your emotional chart, you can get a clear picture of what you might ask for. But asking for what you want won't always get you what you want. If Latoyan's husband no longer felt love for her, then he would not be able to honestly say he loved her. If you want your partner to admit he is emotionally immature, he may deny it vehemently. If you want her to say she never had feelings for the other guy, she might disappoint you with the answer. But if you don't ask for what you want, then you will have an empty space inside of you that will be left unfulfilled. At least hearing an answer that you didn't want is better than hearing no answer at all.

Part of the process of asking for what you need is to figure out what you are ready to hear. In the previous chapter, I described a client who didn't want to hear any details about the affair, for fear she would be forced to take some action to maintain her integrity. One husband I treated knew of his wife's affair but chose not to confront her because he wanted to spare *her* integrity, reasoning, "If I can get the marriage back on track without her ever knowing that I uncovered her affair, then I won't have to make her uncomfortable discussing it."

Everyone's needs unfold at different rates. The risk of asking for too much too fast is that you may not be emotionally strong enough to deal with the response. So, before asking, think through how you will deal with the answer when you get it. If you think you can't process it without resorting to detective work, judgment, or being overwhelmed by emotions, then put it out on the back burner as something to be dealt with later.

Be a conduit, not a roadblock, for conversation

The traumatic impact of discovering an affair stirs up a lot of emotion, much of it negative, and much of it directed toward the perpetrator— your spouse. That's one reason why it is so difficult to have fruitful conversations with this person: he or she is the cause of your pain. You may see it as a tall order to sit calmly during a conversation, but, if you think about it, what choice do you have? When you escalate negativity, it just shuts down further dialogue and brings you further away from your goal of resolution.

Keeping in mind your aim to work toward progress in the relationship, you can help grease the wheels of conversation by maintaining a dialogue and not permitting it to shut down prematurely. One technique is to ask open-ended questions. Rather than ask, "Did you ever think about how I felt during this?" which requires a yes or no answer, ask instead, "What were you thinking my feelings were when this was going on?" (Remember to listen to the answer without judgment.)

You can also keep dialogue open by talking about your partner's favorite subject: himself (or herself). You laugh? Almost without exception, people like talking about themselves. Salespeople use this technique all the time; when you next take a trip to buy a car, notice how the salesperson asks you all about yourself. It's a way of making you feel comfortable and trusting. Keeping the spotlight of discussion on your partner is certain to make it easier for the talks to continue. You may start to feel frustrated when you hear sentence after sentence start with the word, "I," but it's a way to loosen the vocal cords. Remember, also, that people feel more connected to others who listen to them talk about themselves.

When you hear what's on your partner's mind, you may also have an opportunity to learn things you didn't know before and that may help you make sense of the affair. At some point you, too, will need to talk about yourself, but if you do it too early, before your mate is ready to listen, the conversation will shut down as quickly as a Broadway flop.

Another way to assure smooth conversation (beyond letting your mate talk) involves making sure that your partner feels heard. In chapter 11, I will review good listening skills, but for now keep in mind that the best way for someone to feel understood is if you repeat back what they say, sometimes even using their own words. If they say, "I felt confused when I had two commitments at once," your response should be "So, it sounds like you are saying that having two commitments at the same time was confusing." (Even though you're tempted to say, "I should be your first, your last, your every commitment!") When people feel listened to, they are much more likely to listen back. You, also, will want to be heard when your time to speak arrives.

❧ FOR BOTH OF YOU

Keeping the conversation going

A discussion about infidelity, particularly when you converse about it in the context of how you feel about the marriage, is a tough thing to get started, and it's tougher still to keep going. Be sure of one thing, though: maintaining an ongoing dialogue is a necessary part of healing. It is fundamental in reconnecting with your partner and in rebuilding a bond between you.

You know from your dating days how much time the two of you spent talking. Even if you're the strong-but-silent type or the we-never-talked-about-feelings-in-my-family type, when you two first met, much of your time was spent chatting with each other. Whether during a drive, sitting at a bar or restaurant, or taking a walk in those days, it didn't seem like hard work keeping a conversation alive. In fact, talking was how you got to know each other.

Now that your marriage has been rocked by infidelity, it's time to go back to basics. I say this because one of the first things that a victim of infidelity tells me is "I thought I knew this man" or "I thought I knew this woman." The affair tells me that there are things still to be understood between the two of you, and spending time together is the key to doing this.

If talking together after the discovery of an affair sounds tough to do, you're right. But research tells us that there are certain good ways to talk and that following guidelines can smooth the way for easier and more meaningful conversations.

From the Web: Good to Have My Best Friend Back

I have been married for sixteen years. At various times in our marriage my wife has felt that I was a little distant and wanted to be closer to me. She felt I didn't open up to her very much, which was true. I was a little clueless, and I didn't think anything needed to change because I was happy.

Lately I feel like things are reversed, like she is a little distant and I really want to be closer to her. The other night we really opened up to each other and we talked for hours, something we haven't done for years, if ever.

Afterward, she told me "It's good to have my best friend back." It was great. We felt so close to each other.

Set aside time to talk

It's easier to have a meaningful conversation when you know that's what is expected of you. You may have in mind that folding laundry together is a good time to talk, but if your partner doesn't know that, you'll walk away after fifteen minutes with a basketful of folded sheets and an empty heart. If you plan in advance, then you both know that it's time to fire up the vocal cords. You might choose to place it in your schedule days in advance, or you may want to announce to your partner your desire to talk at a certain moment.

Try to be thoughtful about the time of day or the amount of stress that your partner is under at a particular time. Sometimes couples with young children who pick times late in the day are too exhausted to make use of a heart-to-heart conversation. Other couples may spontaneously decide to talk in the middle of the night, when one, or both of them, can't sleep. Sometimes couples have their most fruitful conversations in the wee hours of the night, but just as often the conversation either leads to frustration because one partner keeps falling asleep, or because the dialogue leads to feeling wide awake, and no one can return to sleep. I recommend couples try to avoid the middle-of-the-night talks.

When you feel ready to talk, extend an invitation. Please keep in mind that just because you want to talk at a certain moment doesn't mean your partner wants to. It's best to approach your partner saying, "Honey, I'd like to schedule some time to talk." You and your mate can choose a time within the next day or two. Once you have decided on a when and where, write it on your calendars. If you carry cell phones, use the calendar or alarm function on your phone to set up an alarm to remind you. If you make a commitment to show up for a talk, you must show up. Think about it as you would a business meeting or an appointment with your child's pediatrician. You must make every effort to attend.

What if you need to talk about something that just can't wait? If there is a critical issue that you feel you must be heard on, then it's fair to ask for an emergency talk time. The partner who receives the request must do everything in his or her power to comply with that request. If, however, one partner tends to view *every* need as an *urgent* need, then you must have a conversation about how to define an emergency.

Have time you don't talk

Also be careful about making all "free time" into "talk time." While one of you might enjoy using every last unstructured moment of the day to fit in an extra word or two, the odds are the other secretly (or not so secretly) dreads it. If the "avoider" wants to avoid talking, and the "seeker" uses every opportunity to chat-up the avoider, the avoider will spend less and less time in the company of the seeker, just to steer clear of those extemporaneous conversations. Seekers should be respectful that avoiders need space; just because they don't want to talk as much as the seeker doesn't mean they don't care.

Set time limits on talks

One of the greatest worries of the conversation avoider is that conversations will "never end." Of course, they must end sometime; people do need to sleep or go to work, after all. But, it's as important to set an end time to dialogues as it is to make a start time. A preplanned duration of the discussion will go a long way to helping each participant feel like he or she knows what to expect. By adding structure to the talk you provide a way for each partner to set a pace for the discussion and to maintain better control of the emotions that crop up. I usually recommend that important conversations last about twenty minutes to a half an hour. As you get more practiced at it, you'll be able to schedule longer talks.

An end time doesn't mean that a topic can never be revisited once you're done talking for the day; on the contrary, you should agree that if you haven't completed a subject, you can come back to it on a future talk.

While an end time assures the talk doesn't go on forever, it also serves the opposite purpose, to make sure the talk goes on long enough. On occasion, when emotions run high, one or the other of you may be tempted to throw your hands in the air and give up on the conversation just moments after it begins. Sometimes it's a good idea to give yourself some time away from a heated conversation. But at other times, leaving the room reflects poor communication skills. Knowing that the conversation will last a set period of time will encourage you to stay with it, even though it may be tough. It will improve your communication skills during this difficult time and into the future.

Distinguish between "talk with" and "talk at"

I love the scene from the TV series *Friends,* when Ross meets his girl-friend, Janice, at the coffee shop. She has a serious look on her face, as she announces, "Ross, we need to talk." Ross eagerly responds to the invitation by jumping on the couch, leaning back, and settling in for a long discourse. "Okay," he begins, "Sometimes I feel . . ." After these first words Janice looks at him in annoyance, saying, "No!" She makes it clear that when she says, "We need to talk" what she really means is, "I'm going to talk!" I love that scene because it rings true: too often when one person asks for a "talk" it means they want to talk *at,* not *with,* the other person. That's okay some of the time. But for conversations to progress, you have to be willing to listen as well as talk. Earlier in the chapter, I discussed listening skills, and we will look at them in depth in the next chapter. For now, just keep in mind that if setting up conversations means that you plan to talk *at* your mate, he or she will soon start to cringe whenever you say, "We need to talk."

When possible, touch

I know it's hard on the tail of an affair to hear advice about making physical contact. But touch is one of the strongest ways that humans communicate with each other. By making light contact, you reduce the physical stress for both of you. It's also a way to make sure that there's not too much distance between you. The purpose of talking, after all, is to understand each other better and to grow closer. By bridging the distance between you, you give the message that you are working toward a shared goal.

Boot up your computers

Ten years ago, I was introduced to a novel way of resolving marital discord. I treated a young professional couple in their early thirties who, during a particularly rocky time in their marriage, decided to communicate via e-mail. According to the couple, "Whenever we were in the same room, the tensions got too high." By constructing e-mails to each other, they could proofread their words before they clicked the Send button, and they could take their time responding to e-mail, too. It worked for them, and, while it seemed novel to me at the time, each year more and more couples turn to electronic communication to extend a conversation. Texts are a briefer way of e-mailing; instant messaging is more immediate.

Electronic communication is a good alternative for couples who get flooded with emotion when they talk, for individuals who feel physically threatened by their spouse, or for people who just sense they can't keep up with the pace of their partner's words. It's also the best mode of "talking" for couples who are living apart, particularly military families. These modes of interaction help you to have a dialogue, while removing some of the obstacles to listening and being heard. If you are not geographically separated, then it may be a useful tool (but not the only tool) for conversing. Outside of the e-world, being in the same space, making eye contact, and touching are all modes of communication that can weigh just as heavily as words.

If you do choose to use the electronic option for sharing feelings, take into account a few key principles. Even though you send a message and mark it urgent doesn't mean that your spouse is free, or able, to look at it the second you send it. Sitting by your iPhone waiting for a response will just increase your anxiety and weaken your efforts to improve your marital bonds. If you want direct feedback, schedule a face-to-face. Also, be considerate of your partner's communication style and attention levels. I've read a few five-page e-mails, to which a partner responds in two sentences. It's easy to assume that the partner who writes less cares less, but it's not necessarily so. If you're writing too much, it might make you feel better, but there's a good chance that your partner is going to miss some important points that are buried in the body of the text. In most cases, it's best to keep the communication limited to one printable page.

♣ CROSSING THE BRIDGE

Nobody enters into a marriage wanting to go through infidelity. On top of the terrible emotional torment of discovering the affair, you must deal with unraveling all the details of the affair and the repercussions that follow. Many people wish they could magically just put it all behind them. I wish, for you, there was some other way of getting to the other side of this experience without feeling any pain. But it's just not possible. I don't know if it's worth telling you that one day you will look back at these travails and recognize that you have grown from it and learned from it. Deep down, I suspect you know it's true. After all, you can't help but get something out of it, given the extraordinary amount of effort you have put into it.

I applaud you for your patience and persistence, both you who have been the victim of an affair and you who have chosen to work with your partner after you strayed. By discussing how you feel, and taking the time to listen to how your partner feels, you've taken a big step toward mending the rift in your marriage. In the next chapter, we'll look at how healing the wounds of infidelity will require heartfelt remorse from the person who committed adultery and an opportunity for his or her partner to grant forgiveness.

8

Forgiveness

HAVING A GOOD CONVERSATION with your spouse is priceless. You will grow close in ways that you could never have predicted. There's a lot to talk about, and you may talk for hours on end. Sooner or later your conversation will turn to the topic of forgiveness. Now what?

Take a moment and think about forgiveness. What's it for?

Apologies have to do with our very human penchant to project a future for ourselves and an equally human tendency of others to project a future for themselves that differs from our own. When those two individuals' desires intersect, at least one person's expectations are thwarted. This allows for an apology to take place.

Two people walk through a narrow doorway, each one visualizing going through the door, a split second from now, unencumbered. When they collide, it's obvious that each person's plans interfered with the other's. Typically, they would briefly apologize to each other for bumping shoulders, and go on their way.

Sometimes self-righteousness plays a role in contrasting desires. Say you go to the supermarket wanting to quickly pick up a loaf of bread.

As you enter the checkout line, the guy ahead of you has twenty items in the "twelve items or fewer" lane. He is responsible for impeding your goal of a speedy trip at the supermarket. He, too, had a goal of getting out quickly—that's why he didn't take the regular line. Here the collision of goals requires no apology from you: you followed the rules. What you want is for someone, either the checkout cashier or the checkout line bandit, to acknowledge that you have been inconvenienced by someone who broke the rules. How about an apology right about now?

The principles of apology include

1   One person (or people) has a sense of what ought to happen (based on a specific promise, preconceived notions, or social norms),

2   another person (or people) interferes with that person's expectations,

3   that other person must recognize that he or she had done something (or failed to do something) that impacted that person, and,

4   recognizing that he or she has impeded the goals of that person, the other person should assume liability and, in some discernible way, let the affected person know that he or she takes responsibility for the effects of the action.

1. *One person has a sense of what ought to happen.* In marriage, you have desires concerning what a marriage should be like, and you envision a future based on these desires. Even if you're not one of those people whose closets are organized by colors, or who creates a spreadsheet of your annual projected household expenses, you still have a general vision of what the relationship of marriage will look like. Your expectations might consist of some of these items:

Live in the same home
Talk to each other regularly about hopes and dreams
Have children together
Raise children the same religion
Share bank accounts
Decorate the house for the holidays

These examples are but the tip of the iceberg when it comes to the expectations that people have when they get married. Some of them, such as living in the same home, crystallize when couples cosign on a home mortgage. Others are theoretical, since some couples promise each other that they will have children and then find they aren't able to. Some plans, such as decorating together, remain unspoken, since most people don't talk about every single detail before the wedding.

Other promises that you made to each other were more formal. Wedding vows often include the promise to "love, honor, comfort, and cherish her/him from this day forward, forsaking all others, keeping only unto her/him for as long as you both shall live." It doesn't matter whether you and your bride or groom repeated these exact words or not, for most people a marriage is, above all, a commitment to monogamy.

2. *Another person interferes with that person's expectations.* You may not be able to realistically plan on having a problem-free trip to the supermarket, but when your partner stands in front of your assembled friends and family and promises not to have an intimate romantic relationship with anyone but you, you *ought* to be able to count on that promise. This holds equally true if you and your partner have made a formal promise to each other to date each other exclusively.

Engaging in sexual relationships, emotional affairs, inappropriate intimacy (either live or online), or meaningful continuous relationships outside of the knowledge of a partner—all may cross the bounds of expected behavior of a loyal spouse.

We've spoken about the feelings of hurt and betrayal that such acts stir. What should the unfaithful partner do about it? We've addressed his or her need to end the relationship. We've reviewed the need to answer questions about the affair. We've touched on the need to communicate together as a couple. Now we'll talk about accountability and apologies.

When an affair happens, two of the four principles of apology are automatically met: first, one person has expectations of fidelity from the other based on a promise, and, second, the spouse betrayed that person's expectations. Yet these conditions alone will not prompt the unfaithful mate to believe that an apology is due, despite everything the partner has been through. Why not? Because the person who betrayed the trust must recognize that he or she has broken a promise. Let's look at this for a moment.

3. That other person must recognize that he or she had done something that impacted the person. A highly successful marketing executive was seeing me for relationship help. Melissa had been married once before, and it hadn't worked out. Now she had built a house together with a boyfriend of seven years who constantly described anxiety about committing to marriage. When she found out that he had recently begun to send money to an old high school sweetheart, he responded to her complaints by denying there was anything wrong with helping out an old friend, and that he had done nothing to interfere with Melissa's expectations of him. When, later, he began to see his ex-girlfriend and actually rented an apartment for her, he again stated that there was no expectation, implied or otherwise, that he refrain from doing such a thing. He did not apologize, and, despite a messy financial untangling of her co-joined home, Melissa ended her relationship with this man.

If your mate has made a commitment to fidelity (usually through wedding vows) and has had sex with someone outside of the marriage, then it would seem impossible for your mate not to recognize that he or she has broken a promise. Nonetheless, there are many who, caught red-handed in an affair, plead innocent. Here are some reasons people give to explain why they should not be held accountable for crushing the dreams of their spouse:

- "I never made a formal promise of fidelity, so officially what I did was not cheating."
- "I never crossed the line and had vaginal intercourse with the person; therefore I never broke the promise of fidelity."
- "You left me no choice (either by ignoring my sexual or emotional needs, or by having performed some unfaithful act against me). I had to have an affair to get what I needed, since I couldn't get it through the marriage."

Readers of this book appreciate that there are many kinds of infidelity and that most of the rationales or excuses used to explain these transgressions are just that: rationales and excuses. To the person who has had an affair: in all likelihood, if your partner thinks you've reneged on your promise, then you probably have, even if you believe that your actions were not designed intentionally to hurt anyone. The liability doesn't rest in your intent; it rests in the results of your action. Even if you weren't clear on what the rules were about maintaining fidelity, you do not have an excuse for avoiding the consequences of hurting your spouse.

To the person who has been the victim of an affair: one of the reasons your spouse may not feel the need to apologize is that he or she does not feel that any promises have been broken. Quite possibly, in their mind, your idealized future ("I will have a spouse who will not stray") and their actions ("What I did was not a betrayal") are not incompatible. Just because you see it one way doesn't mean that your spouse sees it the same way.

It's frustrating to think that something so crystal clear to you is so murky to your partner. Keep in mind, though, that although you're committed to a life together, you're not committed to a life of perceiving things the same way. You don't see eye-to-eye in lots of instances, and, while this particular issue carries more significance than whether you prefer chunky or smooth peanut butter, your mate still believes that your interpretation of things is wrong. You can't strong-arm someone into believing what you do. Cajoling, yelling, or threatening won't get your partner to change an opinion. Only through open discussion, in which you make your expectations clear and get a clear picture from him or her as to whether there has been any transgression, will you help your partner to see it through your eyes. (Or, these discussions may help you see that your assumptions of infidelity may have been incorrect. It's possible.)

4. *The other person should assume liability and in some discernible way let the affected person know that he or she takes responsibility for the effects of the action.* This is what it all boils down to. When a person is the cause of your shattered dreams, that person can, and should, apologize. Erving Goffman, one of the twentieth century's most influential experts in social psychology, stated: "Whether one runs over another's sentence, time, dog, or body, one is more or less reduced to saying some variant of 'I'm sorry.'"

From the Web: Forgive and Forget

It's hard to forgive and forget when you catch your wife cheating. The more so when she's not open about it or sorry when she knows you saw it.

—Monty, 35, married eight years

♣ APOLOGIZE

In the pages that follow I talk about the concept of apology. Since the subject of this book is infidelity, and up until now I've led you to appreciate that the person who has had an affair must accept responsibility, you can assume that when I write about how to apologize, I'm talking to that person. Yet everyone who reads this section can learn something. At some point in your life—and probably at many points every day—there will be opportunities to express regret for what you have done to another, either on purpose or by accident. If you're human, you'll need to apologize at some point, so both of you should be sure to read these recommendations and put them to use.

The apology is a complicated form of communication; some researchers have spent years researching all aspects of it. I have broken down the process to five steps:

1 Be genuine.

2 Acknowledge the other's pain.

3 Ask for forgiveness.

4 Offer retribution.

5 Forgive yourself.

Step 1: Be genuine

A genuine apology sounds easy to do. You probably know by now that it's not. I'll bet that on many occasions you've already tried to say, "I'm sorry!" You may also have resorted to the tried and true, "I've already said I'm sorry. What else would you like me to do?" Am I right?

If up to this point you have not once uttered an apology, then offering an apology—"I am sorry"—would be a great place to start. Your mate may not accept the apology the moment you offer it, however. Why? Because it does not feel genuine. Even if, in your heart of hearts, you swear you mean it, it may not be perceived that way. I'd like to help you make sure that your mate knows that you offer a genuine apology.

Before offering the apology, you've got to do a fair amount of introspection to figure out what you are apologizing for.

Own up: If you think you are apologizing for "having an affair," then think again. Above all, you are apologizing for your actions. There is a lot more that you have done, or not done, that led to this affair, and your mate wants you to acknowledge and take responsibility for all of it.

Here are some examples:

- Taking time away from the family to be with the other person
- Lying about where you were and what you were doing
- Potentially embarrassing your spouse in the eyes of his or her friends, family, or neighbors
- Having sex with your partner after you had sex with someone else, potentially increasing risks of sexually transmitted infections
- Breaking your wedding vows
- Contributing to your mate's becoming depressed

There are probably dozens of consequences that could be added to this list; before you stand in front of your mate, you'd better figure out the full extent of your wrongs. What were all the ways that your affair constituted lying? What kinds of deceptions did you engage in? What effect did it have on your children? How did it impact your religious community? Did you use family money for the cost of the affair? You've got to take a good long critical look at yourself. You won't be ready to say you're sorry until you know what you are sorry for.

This may hurt, but in order to help you clear the air, I'll ask you to write down all the ways in which your acts impinged on your spouse. There may be many more people you owe an apology to, but for now, let's focus on that one person you made a lifetime commitment to and take an honest look at how you may have hurt him or her.

No, I mean it. I really want you to sit down with a pen and paper (or keyboard and monitor) and write a list of the things you are sorry for. So go, write, and come back to this part of the chapter when you've completed your list.

Now that you have this list in hand, you are better prepared to offer a genuine apology. So, do you give the list to your mate and say, "Here, honey, this is the stuff I did wrong. Sorry about all that. All set now?" Ummm, no. Not quite.

Speak up

Your partner needs to hear, in your words, what you have done. Saying "I hurt you by my actions" is a start, but your mate needs to know that the thing you are apologizing for is the thing that he or she is hurt by. You have a duty to reveal all the whos, whats, wheres, and hows of your mistakes.

You need to offer your apology with the seriousness and sense of purpose you would anything of this magnitude. This should not be done as an aside while you try to juggle household chores or as you are about to depart on a long business trip or military deployment. It shouldn't be thrown in haphazardly into another conversation. It should be done in a quiet space, with time to process and discuss. It should be done with face-to-face contact whenever possible.

Accept responsibility

When it comes time to offer an apology you must, above all, be clear about what you have done and be absolutely certain not to shirk by sharing the blame with anyone or anything else. Apologizing is not saying. "It never would have happened if I hadn't been drunk," or "If he hadn't come on to me, I wouldn't have gone with him." In particular, be careful to avoid labeling your partner as responsible, as in, "If only I had been getting more love from you, I wouldn't have looked elsewhere." You must present in clear language what you have done, and then take full responsibility for it. You'll know you're on the right track when no one offers any disagreement about what you are apologizing for.

People sometimes try to decrease their own responsibility by apologizing for the other person's reaction to them by adding "if." Saying, "I'm sorry if what I did made you upset" is much different from saying, "I'm sorry for what I did, and I know it upset you." The "if" statement tells the person that you have remorse about the outcome, not about your actions. Don't do that.

Offer alternatives

You've probably heard the advice to stay away from the "coulda, shoulda, woulda" attitude toward life. Well here's a place where this is exactly the attitude you need. A hearty dose of "I should have called you the minute I got in the situation" or "I wish I would have been smart enough to avoid going to that bar" tells your partner that you understand that there "coulda" been a better way of handling things and gives hope that you will make better choices in the future.

Abolish expectations

Another aspect of genuine apology is to offer it without expectation of what you get back. This isn't a proposition of "I'll say what I did wrong so you will tell me what you did wrong" or even "I'll say I'm sorry if you say you forgive me." Your sole goal should be to make sure that your partner hears you. It's certainly all right to offer the hope that your partner will accept the apology, but that cannot be a condition for offering it.

Say "I'm sorry"

You may be thinking you are sorry, very sorry. You may have admitted to all your wrongdoings. You may have asked forgiveness, and promised never to do it again. But, if when it's all done your mate looks at you and says, "But you never said you were sorry," then you didn't say you were sorry. If you are sorry, don't forget to say it.

As an aside, studies (not related to affairs) about gender difference in apology reveal that women tend to offer spontaneous apologies more than men do. Women are more likely to perceive things they have done as requiring the offer of apology, but men tend to see real and even imagined wrongs as not deserving an apology, because they weren't that big of a deal. But in the case of affairs, both sides need to be willing to say they are sorry.

Step 2: Acknowledge the other's pain

You've done wrong. By this time I think everyone's on board with that. We've also acknowledged that you've got to have a clear picture of your transgressions and be willing to accept your responsibility. But an apology doesn't hit home until you are able to also acknowledge the effect it had on the other person. Suppose, on the way to the parking lot after buying your loaf of bread, you see a sports car slam into your minivan. Imagine the driver jumps out of his sports car, runs over to you, and says, "Whoa! I sure did pull out fast, and I didn't look, either. I'm a lousy driver today. Sorry." Afterward he tips his cap, waves ta-ta, and jumps into his car and drives away. Something's missing from that equation. You would want the other driver to take the time to look over your car, and, moreover, to acknowledge that the new dent on your car is a consequence of his actions. He didn't just screw up; his screw-up resulted in a dent in your car. His actions affected you.

When you cheated on your partner, it demonstrated that you did many things wrong and you'll have to spell them out. But accepting responsibility only works if it goes hand in hand with the heartfelt recognition that your actions have harmed your mate. In Step 1, you listed all the ways in which your actions were hurtful. Time to take out the list again and write down all the negative feelings that your act has stirred up in your spouse. He or she will have told you about some of them already. Some, you may be able to extract from chapter 7, which addresses the emotional impact of an affair. You may have to guess at some of the other emotions. In this case, be prepared to have an unfinished list, or even an incorrect list. If you make an effort, your mate will appreciate that you are trying to understand how events traumatized him or her.

At first, you won't be able to distill all the effects of the affair on your partner; your efforts will be incomplete but they will still be very much appreciated. Be ready to listen to more details about the negative impacts of the affair. Your partner is like the owner of a smashed-up car: now that you've accepted that, yes, I did quite a bit of damage, he or she is going to point out every inch of dented and scratched metal so you know exactly what you did wrong. When your partner has pointed these hurts out, add them to the list without getting defensive or judgmental. It will help you with the next step: asking for forgiveness.

Step 3: Ask for forgiveness

Later in this chapter, I'll be talking to your spouse about forgiveness. Here, I'm talking to you. If you have had an affair, you cannot decide whether your partner will forgive you. But you can ask.

Your actions hurt your partner, but unless you have antisocial personality disorder, you feel awful for putting your partner through what you did. Many unfaithful spouses feel racked with guilt for what they have done. If you've become wretched in the aftermath of the affair, it would be such a relief for your partner to forgive you. When one partner forgives the other, it can result in a deep sense of relief for both parties. But just because it would be a relief doesn't mean that it will happen on your timetable, if it happens at all.

I suggest you ask for forgiveness as a gift that your mate can impart to you.

- You cannot demand it: "Why can't you forgive me already? I've done everything you've asked."
- You cannot try to sweet talk it into happening: "Aww, sugar, you know I'd never do anything like that again. Just tell me you forgive me."
- You cannot negotiate it: "I won't ever complain about your watching football again if you just forgive me."

Asking for forgiveness is an act of humility and vulnerability on your part. It frequently comes at the tail end of an apology, once you have completed the process, and may require spelling out your plans to make amends. It may only be at that point, if at all, that your spouse feels ready to grant absolution. He or she should never feel forced to forgive you. Saying, "I hope that one day you'll be able to forgive me" or "I'd like to ask your forgiveness if that's possible" is a healthy, healing way of speaking that leaves the door open for your partner to withhold clemency. You should not put a time frame on it. Granting forgiveness is entirely in your partner's hands.

If your mate has not pardoned you, you may be tempted to check in with him or her regularly. I counsel against that. You were heard, loud and clear; now allow your partner to make some room for his or her heart and emotions to knock it around a little. He or she may become hostile or tearful or shut down completely and not talk for a while. Be patient. Heaven knows your spouse was.

In the Rough

Tiger Woods, in his public apology: "As Elin pointed out to me, my real apology to her will come not in the form of words; it will come from my behavior over time."

Step 4: Offer retribution

This much you know from your own life experience: if someone has done you wrong, you want that person to make it right in some way. That includes saying "I'm sorry," and "I've hurt you," but beyond that, you quite naturally want that person to make it up to you. When the guy in the sports car recognizes the damage he's done, you expect to see his insurance card and have his company fix the car. That's what retribution is about. It boils down to being able to say, "I know I can never undo what I did, but here's what I plan to do going forward."

There is a broad range of possible means of redress after an affair. Here are some changes you must offer:

- Make a commitment to stay faithful in the future
- Agree to transparency in your interactions with other people
- Commit yourself to talk to your partner if there are potential problems in the relationship, rather than run to a different person
- Find ways to improve your marriage
- If you have been involved in substance abuse or other (non-flame) addiction, get the help you need to quit and maintain yourself addiction-free

Some remedies are tailor-made for your situation or your spouse. You may offer to make it up by going to therapy together. Or you might offer to give up some distraction that interferes with your marriage, such as your weekend regattas up and down the east coast.

Some people offer material forms of penance, such as buying a piece of jewelry or tickets to the NBA playoffs. In these cases, you do not want to be seen as trying to bribe your partner away from his or her convictions. Rather, gifts should be offered as a means of saying, "I will put my heart and soul, and even my wallet, into our relationship because I realize you are that important to me." No one promise, or one offering, can possibly compensate for all the pain you have caused your mate.

Never make pledges you cannot keep. If you fully intend to keep your own cell phone on the sly, then you should not promise transparency. If you commit yourself to improving your marriage, then you don't have the option of bowing out of couples' therapy a few weeks later because you think "We're over that." Your partner is worried that you won't follow through on the changes you promise. If you plan to make retribution, you'd better follow through on your promise. As it is, you already have a credibility problem.

Step 5: Forgive yourself

Apologies are an essential part of healing for the person being apologized to, but also to the person who offers the apology—as part of the process of forgiving himself or herself. When people who have had affairs finally wake up from the intoxicating effects of flame addiction, they are sometimes shocked at the chaos and devastation around them. More than one perpetrator of affairs has come into my office, head in hands, sobbing his heart out, incredulous at how much destruction he has caused. Every step in the process of recovery involves sympathy and understanding, but sometimes the harshest critic of the affair ends up being the person who engaged in it. In the rest of this chapter, I will talk about forgiveness. Even though it is written for your spouse, be sure to read it for yourself as well. Your marriage cannot grow if, even in the face of a partner who grants absolution, you cannot forgive yourself.

🍀 GRANTING FORGIVENESS

If you're reading this book as a victim of an affair, you have been challenged to pursue a step-by-step postmortem of the affair and to talk about its emotional impact. You may feel exhausted by all the demands that have fallen on your shoulders. After all, you didn't ask for this affair to happen, why should you have to work so hard at making things right? But for many people who have been cheated on, the most difficult task is yet to come: granting forgiveness.

A definition

What is forgiveness? The International Forgiveness Institute (yes, there really is such an organization) researched this exact question and concluded: "Forgiveness is a gift freely given in the face of a moral wrong, without denying the wrong. Forgiveness welcomes the wrongdoer back into the human community and frees the injured party to pursue the process of healing."

That profound description will serve you well as you examine how your decision to forgive (or not) affects your marriage. Distilled down to its core, it says that a person makes an intentional choice to turn to good, even though he or she has been wronged and even though the person who has committed the wrong deserves wrath. The word forgiveness includes the word "give;" thus, contrary to the impulse to harbor resentment or seek revenge, it involves a wish to offer love and to better the life of the person who has wronged the other.

These factors all intersect in the context of a spouse who has cheated on another. The person who had an affair crossed a line and stirred up a hornet's nest of negative feelings in the spouse. At one point or another, that mate must decide whether dispensing goodwill when the other's act was so hurtful is even possible. But that's the point, isn't it? If there were no such thing as hurt, there would be no such thing as apology and no need for forgiveness.

Forgiveness exists because people commit wrongs that pain other people. While one part of the process involves freeing yourself from your bitterness and anger, another less obvious part of forgiveness consists of releasing your partner from his or her guilt. You can see how amazingly powerful forgiveness can be.

It's quite possible that you've already forgiven your spouse and are turning to this book for help in rebuilding your marriage. If so, I tip my hat to you. The following discussion may give you more insight into the process and may help you in some of your other relationships.

Forgiveness doesn't come easily

Many individuals come to my office weeks or months (sometimes years) after the affair and, while they've decided to stay together and strengthen their marriage, the one who had been cheated on still has not forgiven the offender.

Why is forgiving so hard to do? Here are some of the most common reasons.

You're still angry

You've been hurt before, but the scope of this event has wounded you more intensely than anything you can remember. And the person who did the damage was supposed to be your biggest ally. So, in addition to pain, you feel betrayed. Most people would have good reason to feel furious about the affair, about the lies, about the disrespect. The list goes on. By saying "I forgive you," you may believe you give your mate the message that you are past your anger.

Why would you want to hold onto rage? Because it's yours. It belongs to you, and no one else can control whether you keep it except you. It feels good to be in control of something, even if that thing is negative and destructive. Asking you to let go of your anger feels like you're being asked to release the one clear emotion that you can recognize. You may worry that if you can't feel anger, you won't feel anything at all.

I'm not a big fan of people holding onto anger. The problem with anger is that it develops a life of its own. It requires an intense amount of emotional energy to sustain and takes its toll on your physical and emotional health. In the words of Nelson Mandela, "Resentment is like a glass of poison that a man drinks; then he sits down and waits for his enemy to die." Only when you choose to let go of anger can you regain control of your life.

You want atonement

Your mate has a lot of making up to do, but he or she is not there yet. Making good strides, maybe, but still a ways away. Until he or she has adequately made amends in all the ways you expect it, you're not willing to grant a pardon.

You treat forgiveness as a trade-off, wherein one party (you) will grant absolution when the other party (your spouse) achieves adequate penance. If your partner has made satisfactory (to you) amends, either through words, deeds, or changes in attitude, then you can feel justified in granting forgiveness.

This presents a difficult bind for each of you. On your end, you surrender your power to forgive based on your feelings or your own emotional growth; it puts the whole onus on your partner to earn your clemency. Your partner, in contrast, may become increasingly frustrated because he or she does not know how to pay you back in a way that will satisfy you.

I do believe that a partner has to earn your respect and your trust and that there must be some movement toward change. But forgiveness should be granted as a gift, not payment, for a spouse who wishes to earn back your love.

You believe you'll be a chump

Part of human nature is sharing and creating a society together that is mutually beneficial for everyone. Another part of human nature is that the strong-willed dominate the weak through just about any means possible. So when your husband or wife comes to you asking for a dispensation, you may see this as another opportunity for him or her to get one up on you. Everyone who has been cheated on knows the saying, "Fool me once, shame on you. Fool me twice, shame on me."

If you choose to forgive, though, you don't have to view it as demonstrating weakness in any way. You have endured much; you can choose to hold on to your negativity and continue to hold a grudge or you can choose to let go. In these times, recall the words of Mahatma Gandhi: "The weak can never forgive. Forgiveness is the attribute of the strong."

You don't want to dilute the crime

You may be afraid that saying "You're forgiven" is like saying, "it's no big deal," or "no harm done." As far as you're concerned, it *was* a big deal, and *lots* of harm was done. You want your partner to know that it was serious and that's why it's so difficult to exonerate him or her.

Forgiving someone does not mean that his or her offenses were not serious. Throughout history, people have forgiven horrible industrial accidents, murders, atrocities, and even genocides. There is a way of saying, "What you did was very serious and hurt me very much" while also granting forgiveness. Finding that way takes a lot of guts, but it's something that eventually you'll need to do if you choose to live a life together—and if you, the hurt party, want to move forward in your life.

You want to inflict punishment

You were hurt, really hurt. And you want to hurt your partner back. You have ruled out having an affair yourself or engaging in physical violence. But one power you have at your fingertips is your power to forgive. Your partner may ache for your clemency, but if you withhold it, you wield great power over him or her. You feel justified because, in your mind, you are simply "giving him/her a taste of his/ her own medicine."

Withholding forgiveness does give you back some control over the situation, and that feels good for a while. But ultimately, having a wounded spouse doesn't make you any stronger and makes the marriage weaker. If each of you is going to make an honest effort at rebuilding the marriage, it has to come from a place of strength: the strength to grant forgiveness.

You don't want it to happen again

You may ask, "If I forgive you, what's to keep it from happening again?" Many people equate forgiveness with saying "It never happened" or "It's all forgotten about." Not speaking words of pardon is like keeping the latch in place on the barn door. These people are afraid that once their partner hears the words "I forgive you," their inappropriate behaviors will come charging out again. And then the injured party will have no control over the situation at all.

The reality is, whether you choose to grant forgiveness or not, you really can't control whether your spouse has an affair. You can control the degree to which your partner feels close to you and the extent to which he or she feels hopeful about a future with you. That's why, for some couples, being able to forgive helps reduce the risk of infidelity in the future.

Moving toward forgiveness

You may have many reasons why, in the face of your partner's apologies, you aren't ready to grant forgiveness. Forgiveness does not imply that you condone a person's behavior or even that you necessarily wish to continue having a relationship with that person. But there are some reasons why granting forgiveness may be the right thing to do for you—such as the following.

You free up your emotional energy

Certain basic essentials are necessary for humans to survive. We require a certain amount of caloric intake, fluids, protective clothing, and shelter from the weather. Once the core needs are met, humans can apply themselves to many creative endeavors. To go beyond basic existence and elevate our quality of life, we need to invest high levels of emotional energy.

When individuals are optimistic and have a positive vision for the future with a sense of competence, they increase their level of creativity and, as a by-product of the positive things that happen from that creativity, they experience even greater pleasures and more energy. Engaging in activities, from completing a crossword puzzle to cooking a new recipe, provides a sense of accomplishment and induces higher levels of a "can-do" attitude. A lighter mood and a greater sense of vigor are the natural results.

In contrast, when you hold on to negative feelings, you deplete your spirit of its energy. You lose the inspiration for finding new and better ways to do things. You can still provide the bare necessities for yourself, but the frills, the whimsy, and the resourcefulness—the elements that helped you grow emotionally—disappear. Holding back on forgiveness and maintaining bitterness rob you of your positive energy, leave you feeling drained, incomplete, and barely getting by.

Your own mental attitude colors the relationship

We constantly communicate our attitudes, everywhere we go, and much of the time we do it unconsciously. When you convey a sense of positivity, upbeat attitude, and a spirit of hopefulness, it elevates the quality of your life and the life of people around you.

It's easy to understand how disappointment, anger, hurt, and resentment can cause a negative transformation in your household. Even if you don't spend the day communicating your level of displeasure and pain verbally, you can be sure that your life partner senses these emotions and that they prevent your home from being infused with positive emotion. If you believe in the transformative power of a positive attitude, then you know what you must do. Through forgiveness, you use your ability to let go of negativity, regain your positive outlook, and bring healthier energy to the home.

You improve your health

Researchers from around the world have taken a careful look at the positive effects that forgiveness can produce in the human body. Negative emotions increase stress hormones and throw off your body's sense of physical equilibrium.

In addition to a greater sense of spiritual and psychological well-being, offering an apology can lower your levels of anxiety and stress, reduce your blood pressure, decrease your risk of having alcohol or other substance abuse problems, and reduce the symptoms of depression.

From the Web: A Discussion on Forgiveness

FloridaLady: Since I found out about my husband's contacts with the other woman, he gave me all passwords, locks, etc. He said he wants to do all he can to rebuild my trust, and that really means a lot. I still feel hurt and scared, but he has really shown remorse and love, and from what I have read, that's so rare. I guess when you give your all in a marriage it's so scary to see, even as innocent as it can be, how easily heartbreaks and mistakes can happen.

Elizacol: Been there, done that, FloridaLady. As the victim of infidelity, the advice I can give you is that your husband did the right thing. Or at least he tried, and is trying, to do the right thing. Many husbands in this situation would not do so.

Your wonderful husband sensed that he was on the brink of an affair and immediately tried to put a stop to it. That speaks volumes. Like Dr. Haltzman states, getting out of a relationship, even a friendship, is not easy. Sounds like your husband tried. As well, he is now being open and honest and is apparently willing to communicate with you. These are all good signs.

I would use those efforts by your husband . . . all of those efforts . . . as tools to help you with your forgiveness. In fact, have you thanked him for his honesty? For his willingness to be open with you? For his truly trying to cut off this friendship? It sounds silly to thank him, but honestly, it is something to thank him for.

No human being is perfect. We all make mistakes. Is one mistake necessarily bigger than another? Perhaps. Or, perhaps not . . .

How to grant forgiveness

Granting forgiveness is your chance to take the future of the relationship into your own hands. I'd like to help you go about it in a meaningful dialogue. First, let's consider the goal of forgiveness. In most cases, the cheating spouse offers an immediate "I'm sorry" to the cheated spouse—sometimes within seconds of uncovering of the affair—and hopes that all will be forgiven in that instant. However, the level of emotional turmoil is so high in the moments right after the affair is discovered that the "mea culpa" is almost meaningless.

Forgiveness is rarely granted in that instant because the person whose life has been turned upside down isn't ready. That makes sense. As painful as it is, the couple must first process the event, and trust must once again be established. That takes talk, and time, and thought.

An apology offered by your other half obtains real meaning when you feel like he or she has regained control of his or her behavior (in other words, stopped messing around with other people) and has recognized the extent to which the affair injured you. Now the ball lands in your court. When you feel like enough trust has built up between you two (this will not be total and complete blind trust— that will take a long time in coming, if ever at all), then accepting the apology, and offering clemency, communicates your willingness to work with your partner to heal the wounds.

Every couple goes through the process of healing differently, and each has their own pace. Knowing how to forgive can be as difficult as knowing how to apologize, so having a road map to follow can really help. Here's what I suggest.

Express your feelings

On the one hand, many people feel so awful about what they have done that they need to talk, and talk a lot, about their actions and their guilt. On the other hand, there are others who, when they seek forgiveness for an offense, ideally hope that you will simply say, "Oh, that! I forgot all about it," or, better still, "It was nothing!" This wrongdoer holds onto an unconscious desire that his or her sins can somehow just disappear from the history books. But you haven't forgotten, and no one who is thinking straight would say that an affair was nothing. When you prepare to forgive someone, you should hear that person out, but just as important, you want to make sure that you tell your partner exactly how *you* feel. This is a good opportunity to use the skills described in chapter 7.

Set the stage by telling your partner that you just want him or her to listen—not respond, and not talk back. You might say, "I would like to forgive you for what happened, but before I do, I need to talk about how it affected me. What I have to say will be very difficult for you to hear. Some of my thoughts may be off base, or you may think they are inaccurate. But these are my thoughts, and it's very important for me to tell you what they are. I'm not offering them for debate, just for you to hear and understand."

You get the full attention of your mate when you start the dialogue implying that it will lead to forgiveness. He or she wants your pardon, and this gives you an opportunity to feel in control of the conversation. In your partner's rush to put things behind you both, this may be your best prospect to feel heard.

This is an excellent chance for you and your partner to use reflective listening skills, and we'll talk more about that in chapter 11. You might say: "Honey, what I am saying feels so important to me that I need to know that you understand what I am saying. It would be nice if you agreed, but that's not what I need most right now. I just need to feel heard. After I say what's on my mind, I'd like to ask you to repeat it back to me, to make sure that I expressed myself accurately. If I don't feel like you heard me quite right, I don't want you to feel offended if I try to restate my point. It's that important to me that I make myself understood."

I know it's a mouthful. Believe it or not, I ask many of my patients to memorize the passage above. You can even read it from the book if you like. This approach gives your partner specific tasks: listen and repeat back. Also, it says that your goal is to express yourself clearly rather than to imply that your partner is a poor listener. You might think that it's unnatural to ask your partner to repeat back what you said, but repetition is a powerful tool for improving communication.

Once you feel your partner understands what you went through and doesn't try to minimize, rationalize, or any-other-ize, then you'll feel ready to move on to the next phase of forgiveness.

Take charge of your emotions

You've told your mate what was on your mind, and it's tempting to ask him or her to do something to fix you. *That only makes sense*, you reason, *because your partner is the one who broke you in the first place.* Your spouse must make significant behavior changes, but it's not his or her job to change how you feel. You're the one who has a responsibility to cultivate your own emotional health. When you can recognize what emotions belong to you (as you did in the previous chapter), you can put them in their place and prepare yourself to forgive.

Part of taking care of you may include practicing stress management techniques, including meditation, prayer, or yoga, or seeking professional help from a therapist or spiritual counselor.

Empathize

One of the most difficult challenges in offering forgiveness is opening yourself up to understanding how your partner feels. We tend to instinctively measure someone else's behavior against what we expect of ourselves. We might say, "I would never do what you did," or "How would you feel if I did that?" But another person's ideas about what's right and wrong, about how to avoid getting into (and how to get out of) messy situations differ from yours. Holding your partner to all your standards might be convenient, but it's not realistic. At the very least, it *is* realistic to expect the standard of not sleeping around with anyone else. I get that. But when you gauge all of your partner's activities against your own measuring stick, it may not be fair to either one of you. One of the best ways to feel peace of mind for yourself (and to get through to someone else) is to genuinely appreciate where that person is coming from. Seeing things through his or her eyes helps you to soften the judgment and be more likely to fully forgive.

Be patient

Since the affair things have not been the same. Even if you and your partner have done everything you could to get the marriage back on track, there will still be a lot of work to move things forward. You may feel that until the potholes are all filled in, you won't be ready to progress to an improved relationship. However, it may take months, sometimes years, to get to the point when you and your partner again feel a close bond to each other. You don't have to forgive the first time you start to feel a connection. But postponing forgiveness until all is healed isn't necessary. You have the freedom to choose to forgive when you feel ready.

Move forward

Once you've told your partner that you have forgiven him or her, you must move on. You've been patient, you've been thoughtful, and you've been clear. You have demonstrated great strength. This is a chance to give relief to your mate and to experience a sense of relief for yourself. Don't blow it by ruminating on the way you forgave him or her, what you might have said, or asked for, differently, what kind of reaction you got, or whether or not your forgiveness was well timed or well placed. Enjoy the gift of the lifting of your anger and resentment.

All along you may have believed that when you forgive, you release your partner. The truth is that when you forgive, you release yourself from holding on to the negative emotion. That clears the way for a lot of good changes in the future. In the next chapters, we'll talk about the kinds of things that happen in marriages that drag you down and what you can do to move forward to enrich your relationship and reduce the risk of infidelity ever entering into your marriage again.

9

What to Expect When You're Expecting (a Happy Marriage)

HOW MANY TIMES HAVE you heard people say, "If someone had an affair, then there must have been problems in the marriage in the first place"? Here's my response to that: "You're right!" There is definitely a problem in every marriage in which infidelity happens. Not only is there a marital problem in every marriage in which infidelity happens, there is a marital problem in every marriage in which infidelity *does not* happen. In other words, every marriage has problems. Some married couples may tell you they have never had a disagreement. Believe me, they have, it's just that they don't remember, because the memory of their arguments have faded over time. Couples who have divorced, of course, can recall many disagreements; they went their separate ways before they could heal over their scars, so they still recall the negatives.

This chapter looks at the root of the most common stresses that affect marriage. In fact, almost everything in this chapter you could expect to find in any book or article I might write about all married couples, not just those who have dealt with infidelity. When you finish reading this chapter, you'll know better how to take next steps toward rebuilding your marriage (which we'll talk about in chapter 11).

Many couples (and therapists) take issue when I talk about core marital problems in the same breath as infidelity. The very mention of "problems that have contributed to the affair" appears to lay blame on the victim. I don't wish to do that, since I'm a firm believer that no matter how bad a relationship is, people who choose to go outside marriage for intimacy hold full responsibility for their actions. I do not see infidelity as a justifiable course of action no matter what problems you're having.

But the correlation of marital satisfaction and fidelity cannot be ignored. If a marriage has enough positive value, then someone is much less likely to leave that marriage. However, if the quality of a marriage is poor, then the couple will be less settled and more likely to roam. Marital problems increase the *need* component of the NOD (the Need, Opportunity, and Disinhibition discussed in chapter 5) and increase the likelihood of having an affair.

But there are other aspects of marital dissatisfaction that are worth commenting on. Let's start by looking at perception. Marital quality may not reflect objective fact but rather the observer's subjective viewpoint. Some marriages may be comfortable enough, happy enough, and rewarding enough until something happens within one of the individuals that changes how the marriage is seen. One of my favorite examples is from Leo Tolstoy's *Anna Karenina*, in which Anna (who in an earlier scene had offered marriage-saving postaffair advice to her sister-in-law) returns home from a train ride during which she flirts with the young, handsome Count Vronsky. As Anna gets off the train, she glances over at her heretofore good-enough husband. Now she stares at him as he approaches her carriage and notices, for the very first time, how his big ears stick out so much that they "prop up the brim of his hat." Anna is "struck by the feeling of dissatisfaction with herself that she experienced on meeting him." Although she had not previously noticed this feeling, "now she was clearly and painfully aware of it."

❧ FAILED EXPECTATIONS

You may find Anna's perception of her husband's shortcomings—big ears—silly in comparison with the ways your mate doesn't measure up (or the ways your mate complains about you). Anna is a literary creation; she's not real life, but there is a quality of authenticity to her lament that touches on almost every relationship. When people begin having feelings of marital displeasure, they start to pay attention to small annoyances. Many of my couples' therapy sessions have focused on complaints ranging from excessively mayonnaised tuna fish sandwiches to five-minute late arrivals for appointments. One 70-year-old woman whom I had seen in couples' therapy was outraged when her (third) husband told his sister not to serve shellfish at a dinner party because his wife didn't like it. "I like shellfish perfectly fine," she informed me, "but I can't eat it because of allergies." She viewed her husband's misrepresentation of her food choices as offensive because they didn't reflect well on her. Thus, trivial, almost inconsequential things become deal breakers.

Most people recognize that small complaints are often representative of bigger issues. Poorly made tuna sandwiches show lack of sensitivity to a husband's needs; arriving late for appointments devalues a wife because it disrespects the importance of her time, and incorrectly describing an allergy as a dislike shows lack of compassion that certain food allergies can even be life-threatening.

Psychoanalysts paint one person's dissatisfaction with another as stemming from deeply hidden needs, impulses, and drives. Even top-notch marriage therapists believe that people unconsciously choose life partners with the unrealistic expectation that the partner will complete some need in them that their parents failed to fulfill. Thus, therapists look at marital disappointment as the result of people repeating these maladaptive patterns from their childhood.

I take a simpler approach. I believe that the very nature of marriage—being in a forever relationship with one mate and one mate only—means that each partner will notice unsavory traits in the other. A person chooses a mate (or, in the case of arranged marriages, someone was chosen for another) with the hope that the mate will have the insight and skill to figure out that person's needs and, furthermore, regularly take action to meet them, even at the expense of meeting his or her own needs. When the mate falls short of these expectations, a person may feel resentful at the lack of skill, insight, or initiative to do what is wanted or needed. That resentment begins a cascade of emotions that often ends in intense hostility toward a partner. At its core, it goes something like this: "If you loved me, you would meet my expectations. You have failed to do so, so that means that you don't love me. If you don't love me it means that you're the wrong person for me." Sometimes this line of reasoning leads to divorce, sometimes to affairs.

From the Web: Relationships Don't Follow a Script

If I had a magic wand, I would ban fairy tales and movies and television, as they are the basis for much of the misconception about who we are and what we should be. We have all been conditioned to believe that our relationships should follow a prescription—and when the script isn't followed, anger and disappointment ensue.

—Cassie, divorced

❧ WHEN PARTNERS' SUPPORT FLOUNDERS

Think about the times you or your partner have said (or thought), "My friends know what I need better than you do" or "My friends stand by me when you don't." These thoughts emerge from an assumption that the *least* your partner ought to be capable of is knowing what you need. Whenever I think about this comparison with friends, I think of what author and marriage therapist Patricia Love says on the subject: "Now, try telling your friends that they are *obligated* for the rest of their lives to stand by you, understand your needs, and provide sympathy and support. Then see what happens." Pat's point (and mine) is that when compassion and understanding are optional, people often provide them willingly and easily. When you have a handful of friends, one or two might feel "not in the mood" to discuss your problems. You won't know, though, because they simply will let their phones go to answering machines or they will text back that they're busy. You move on to the supportive friend who is available, and you still see your friends, in general, as being better to you than your own mate.

Another difference between your friends and your spouse is that when your spouse supports your dreams, he or she stands on the receiving end of the consequences. For example, I treated a physician, Ben, and his wife, Sonia. As their children grew, Ben's full-time medical practice supported Sonia through a number of temporary part-time jobs. When he was reluctant to pay for her to open a spa, she accused him of not supporting her dreams and he agreed to provide the funds. Two years later, with close to a hundred thousand dollars invested, Sonia decided that she no longer wanted to run a spa, and she shut it down. The following year, she began receiving applications for law school in the mail and was upset when Ben did not demonstrate excitement over the prospect of Sonia's desire to be a lawyer. To highlight her disappointment, Sonia pointed out how excited and positive her friends were about her new dreams and accused Ben of "raining on my parade."

Perhaps you side with Sonia on this one, or perhaps you can relate more to Ben. Whether she ended up getting a law degree isn't the issue (Sonia decided to drop the idea when she realized she would have to study for the LSATs). What is at issue here is the strain a marriage experiences when one partner's decisions, lifestyle, or values affects the other in a potentially negative way. If you spend enough time together, eventually every marriage will have times when partners don't see eye-to-eye and each one feels as if the other has not met the bare minimum expectation: to support the other at all times.

It's not just the husband who is subject to a demotion in this scenario. From Ben's perspective, Sonia's appeal could diminish if he sees her as being insensitive to the financial and time needs of the family or if he takes offense at her unfounded condemnation of his character. While her credo becomes: "If he loved me, he would stand by my side in enthusiastic support no matter what I say. That's what my friends do," his version of marital strife would be expressed as: "The right woman for me wouldn't keep stressing me out with her pie-in-the-sky dreams, and then get pissed at me for being the sensible one in the family."

Over the course of couples' treatment, Ben and Sonia discussed many occasions when one or the other did not feel supported in the marriage. Was this couple doomed to marital failure? Absolutely not. I was able to help Ben and Sonia understand each other. The part of therapy that most helped save this marriage was clarifying the couple's expectations. Disagreeing with each other, and, yes, at times not supporting the other, happens in every marriage. It's normal.

❧ DEFINING EXPECTATIONS

Supporting dreams for the future is one expectation, and so is appreciating the financial and emotional needs of a family and how your personal plans will affect them. Whether it's preparing meals, being on time, distinguishing between true medical conditions and simple food dislikes, and a million other facets of marriage, you have expectations. Most of these expectations, by the way, were formed before you ever met your mate. When was the last time you put down in writing what those needs were? To move forward in resolving marital discord, I ask you to begin to keep track of the things you look to your partner to bring to the marriage table. This will require a sharp pencil, an open mind, and a fair amount of your time.

In the first column of the chart on the next page you will list all the things that you expect from marriage (or, more specifically, from your partner in marriage). Include your hopes from before the wedding vows were shared to this very day. Consider all the aspects of

Expectations from my partner

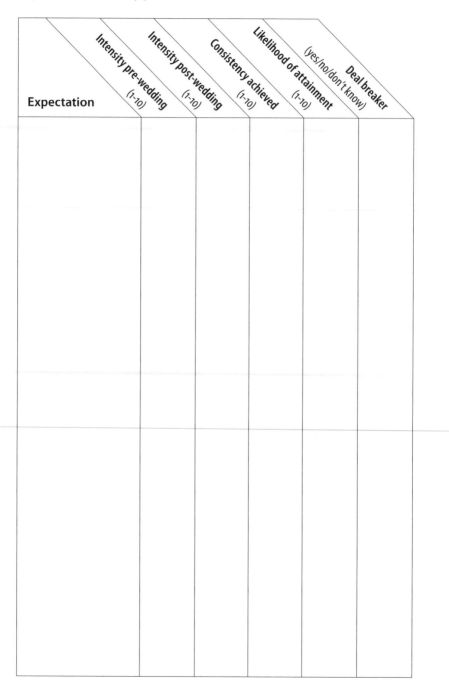

Expectation	Intensity pre-wedding (1–10)	Intensity post-wedding (1–10)	Consistency achieved (1–10)	Likelihood of attainment (1–10)	Deal breaker (yes/no/don't know)

your mate's behavior that you believe ought to be part of the marital package. You can run the gamut, from "sex whenever I want it" to "always hold the door open for me." Include mandatory attendance at religious functions, if that's important to you, or a prohibition against picking teeth within your sight. You'll find that once you start writing down your expectations, more will come flooding to you. Wash dishes? Write it down! Call before coming home from work? Deposit his or her paycheck into a joint account? Put ink to paper.

The more expectations you can think of, the more helpful this exercise will be, *but,* before you start filling in the first column, let me impart a few words of caution. First, I am aware that you are reading this book because infidelity has had an impact on your life, and it's hard to get the infidelity out of your head. But this exercise is not just about infidelity. It's tempting to write about five hundred legitimate expectations regarding proper behavior regarding your mate's interactions with attractive others—everything from "Never pick up a voice mail from the affair mate" to "Don't lie to me about your whereabouts." These are fair expectations, but the focus here is broader. It goes beyond fidelity-related issues.

Next, be as specific and action-oriented as possible. Think to yourself: "If someone were taking a video of my mate would they be able to see him or her achieving the goal?" For instance, "Have an emotional connection" is too difficult for you or your partner to measure. How will you or your partner know when this prospect is met? Rather, using a more specific expectation, such as "Will sit by my side when I talk about my emotions" would result in an observable standard that your mate may or may not achieve. Another example of vague expectations is "Treat me with respect." Consider instead, "Ask me questions about my opinions and thoughts," "Refrain from using off-color language," or some other way that would spell "R-E-S-P-E-C-T" when you see it.

Also, when people do this exercise, they tend to focus on their unmet needs. People will rush to write "Buy me flowers weekly" when they are not getting flowers, but they forget to write down

"Pick up laundry on the way home from work" when it is getting done regularly. Also partners will list "Eat healthy" when their mate is overweight but will neglect to add, "Work out regularly" when they have a fit partner. This is a list of your expectations, not your complaints (although, as you will see, there is quite a bit of overlap). So be sure to include things that are happening regularly if they are important to you.

Okay, ready to start? Go to the chart, fill in the first column, use extra paper if you need to, and check back in with me when you are done.

If you really let yourself be creative on this one, you went well past the space allotted, and, once you came up for air, realized that you could probably have listed dozens more expectations.

Whenever my patients do this exercise, I am reminded of a wonderful book by Lori Gottlieb called *Marry Him: The Case for Settling for Mr. Good Enough*. Part autobiography, part investigative reporting, and part *Millionaire Matchmaker*, the book takes the premise that young women are too selective and often pass up good enough husbands in the search of a better variety. She begins her book with a list of "must haves" for her future husband. Below is only a partial list of the characteristics that Lori expects from the man of her dreams:

- Intelligent
- Kind
- Extremely funny
- Curious
- Loves kids
- Financially stable
- Emotionally stable
- Sexy
- Intuitive
- Generous
- Same religion but not too religious
- Optimistic but not naive

- Ambitious but not a workaholic
- Talented but humble
- Warm but not clingy
- Grounded but not boring
- Soulful but not new-agey
- Vulnerable but not weak
- Quirky but not weird
- Free-spirited but responsible
- Charismatic but genuine
- Strong but sensitive
- Athletic but not a sports nut
- Open-minded but has conviction
- Decisive but not bossy
- Mature but not old
- Flexible but can compromise
- Sophisticated—well-educated, well-traveled, has been around
- Over 5'10" but under 6'0"
- Has a full head of hair (wavy and dark would be nice—no blonds)
- Likes my friends (and I like his)
- Not moody
- Trustworthy
- Is literary and enjoys wordplay
- Likes discussing (but not arguing about) politics and world events
- Stylish
- Stimulating
- Not a slob—respectful of our living space
- Is madly in love with me!

The punch line is that Lori, in her early forties, was still single when she wrote the book. We'll talk about Lori's book later in the chapter, but for now, whatever you have written, even if it is not as exhaustive as Lori's list, is enough. You can always add more later on. Here's an example of how you might start the chart, using two expectations only.

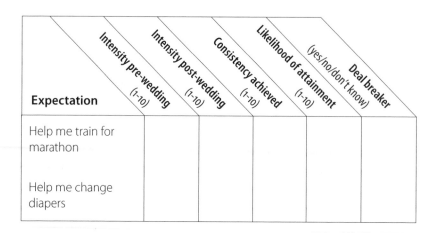

Expectation	Intensity pre-wedding (1-10)	Intensity post-wedding (1-10)	Consistency achieved (1-10)	Likelihood of attainment (1-10)	(yes/no/don't know)	Deal breaker
Help me train for marathon						
Help me change diapers						

How important is that expectation?

In the next column of the chart, on a scale of 1 to 10 (10 being the highest importance), rank the intensity or importance of each of the listed expectations for your husband or wife *before you married* (or before you each committed to a long-term relationship to) each other. For many people, staying faithful would be a 10. However, if when you married you expected your husband to help you train for marathons, though this was not of critical importance, you might rank it a 3. If you expected your husband to help change diapers but you were willing to share the task, you might rank it a 2.

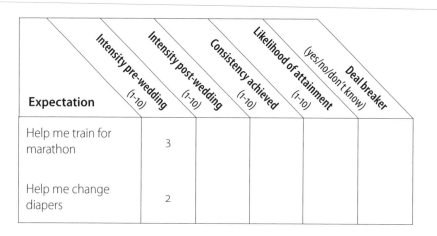

Expectation	Intensity pre-wedding (1-10)	Intensity post-wedding (1-10)	Consistency achieved (1-10)	Likelihood of attainment (1-10)	(yes/no/don't know)	Deal breaker
Help me train for marathon	3					
Help me change diapers	2					

When you've completed the second column, use the same numeric scale in the third column to rank the intensity or importance of each of these expectations *currently.* Expectations like "Stay faithful" usually don't decline in rank. But if you married expecting your husband to stand in the rain with a stopwatch, and in the years since the wedding he decided he'd rather stay dry at home, you may have decided that his participation in your goal is not all that important, and you may lower that number to a 2. If early on in your relationship you didn't plan on working outside the home, but now you are the main breadwinner and your husband is unemployed, your expectations of his changing diapers might now be a 10.

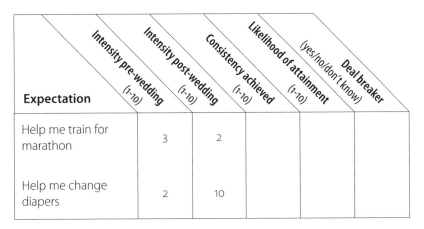

Expectation	Intensity pre-wedding (1-10)	Intensity post-wedding (1-10)	Consistency achieved (1-10)	Likelihood of attainment (1-10)	(yes/no/don't know)	Deal breaker
Help me train for marathon	3	2				
Help me change diapers	2	10				

Spousal report card

Moving on to the fourth column, take some time to assess your partner's success in achieving your expectations. It's easy to see that the diaper-changing husband gets a 10 on this one. But even if he no longer helps time your marathons, he may still help prepare high carb meals on the day before a race or may drive you to a training session. So he earns a 2 or 3, because, while you had expectations that he do much more, he is exerting *some* effort.

Be careful in this column. Most people have an all or nothing attitude about whether someone meets their needs. If you have the hope that your spouse bring home gifts that you like, but he or she has never done so in all the years you have known him or her, you would write a zero. But, is it really true that there was never *one time* when something was brought home that pleased you? A necklace? A jigsaw puzzle? A pizza? A pair of tickets to Monster Truck exhibition? When you think hard about whether someone has ever met your expectations, you realize that your partner may score higher than when you first considered the question. Rather than respond to the gift-giving expectation with 0, consider a rating of 1 or 2.

Before you begin to fill in this column, let's revisit the expectation of "Stay faithful." If you have been the victim of an affair, you may see your spouse as scoring an automatic 0 in meeting this expectation. After all, fidelity is set up as an all-or-nothing proposition—you either cheat on your spouse or you don't. Keep in mind, though, that there are people whose partners have had affairs consistently, even cheating on the day of the wedding. These individuals clearly have not even met the minimal level of expectation for remaining faithful. But think about how loyal your mate has been up until the affair. In my opinion, it should count for something. Consider choosing a score other than 0 if there has ever been sustained fidelity in the marriage.

Now, go ahead and take a stab at filling in the column called "Consistency achieved."

Expectation	Intensity pre-wedding (1-10)	Intensity post-wedding (1-10)	Consistency achieved (1-10)	Likelihood of attainment (1-10)	(yes/no/don't know) Deal breaker
Help me train for marathon	3	2	2–3		
Help me change diapers	2	10	10		

As you go down the list filling in this column, you may discover a disturbing pattern: more often than not your mate has not met your expectations even halfway. Do not despair. If you were to average out the results of your peers, coworkers, and friends, you'd see what I have discovered, that the majority of people are in the same boat, with scores no higher than a 5. But even in couples not affected (or not yet affected) by infidelity, very few people will regard their spouse as providing enough of the attention and appreciation that they deserve. With rare exception, everybody thinks their spouse comes up short. Compared with when they were dating, most people are disappointed with what they're getting in their marriage. I tell you this not to discourage you (and it does seem discouraging) but to help you realize that these feeling may be a normal part of marriage. You are not alone. I'll come back to this later in the chapter.

Can the goal ever be met?

Column five asks you to weigh in on the question of achievability. What is the likelihood that your partner will ever fully meet your expectation? If someone scored a ten on the previous "achievement" score, he or she gets a ten here. If he changes diapers all the time, then it's a pretty sure thing he's got the ability to do it in the future. If your husband used to help you train but has stopped because of children at home, you might look forward to him helping you in the future, so you might put a 4 in the fifth column. Could your husband ever learn to pick out a good present for you? Your first thought is "Hopeless," and you'd be inclined to score a zero.

Here is another area of caution when filling out this chart. People often assume that because a partner has fallen short in the past he or she will continue to fail "to infinity and beyond." That often does happen, but not necessarily because of another person's fault. When people want a certain behavior from someone else, they tend to repeat negative patterns, and then they are frustrated when the same thing happens time after time. Let's use, for example, the ability to pick out the perfect gift for special occasions. Few women have the kind of husband who knows exactly how to buy for them. Imagine a woman pointing to an item in a magazine and saying, "This is pretty" to her hubby six months before her birthday. Then exactly half a year later her husband presents her with that very item neatly wrapped and ribboned, sitting beside her breakfast plate (which, by the way, he set up the evening before). That would be nice, but he would be a rare bird. Many women hint at what they want to their husbands repeatedly and get frustrated birthday after anniversary after Valentine's Day because their husbands never seem to get it right.

♣ TAKING RESPONSIBILITY FOR GETTING WHAT YOU WANT

In my book *The Secrets of Happily Married Women*, I suggest that if wives want a particular present from their husbands, they help their guy succeed in "getting it right." I advise writing a list of what you want, cut out a picture from a magazine, include websites from where your husband can order. I recommend pasting it on his bathroom mirror before your special day or leaving a voice mail at his work, if need be, to remind him. Add something to his calendar on his iPhone, and even snap a photo of it, so it will spring to his attention on the right date.

Of all things I write in the *Happily Married Women* book, this is one of the most controversial. I'll bet (if you're a person who very much treasures gifts but whose mate never picks out the right present for you) you have the same stirrings of controversy inside of you. It goes something like this, "Why should I have to take the initiative to make sure my partner gets this right? Shouldn't he be the one to take responsibility to please me, especially if I tell him what I want? Telling him once should be enough." I understand. And before I became a marriage educator, I would have said the same thing.

You basically feel that once you've let your heart's desire be known, you should be able to sit back and wait for the gifts to come. So I ask you: "How's that plan working out for you?" I've dealt with so many people with chronic frustration over special occasion gifts that I really wonder if setting up the expectation makes the disappointment even worse. Think about the amount of mental effort that goes into hoping for something special. Don't you feel resentful when those hopes aren't realized? Remember what I wrote earlier in this chapter: resentments emerge because your spouse lacks the skill, insight, or initiative to do what you expect. Remember also that resentment often ends in hostility. By suggesting that you go beyond hinting ("Isn't this pretty, honey?") and that you actively make sure that your dreams come true ("Honey, here's a copy of my 'wish list'"), I'm offering a way to reduce your level of resentment and improve your chances of getting what you want.

Here's another suggestion for getting what you want. Buy a gift for yourself, wrap it festively if you like, and give it to your husband on your birthday to give to you. And when he does so, thank him profusely. The point is this: in the end, you will have a gift that you want. And, despite your belief to the contrary, your husband will not feel like he has lost his power in this exchange. Most likely he will feel uplifted because you reinforce the fact that you got a present from him that you really wanted. This helps him meet his expectation of "My wife appreciates my gifts."

By no means am I asserting that men are free of responsibility for getting gifts right. In my book *The Secrets of Happily Married Men,* I recommend specific ways for men to take the initiative for remembering their wives' special days and special needs. The reason I talk here about what women can do, and not men, is because this section uses an example of a wife's expectations. Thus the action plan for the wife is designed to help the husband score better in the "likelihood of achieving" column. If there were a male corollary to a woman's expectation here, it would be a man who wishes that his wife would be pleased with the treats he buys her. You can see how, if this section were focused on meeting that expectation instead, I would be giving a different set of suggestions to a man, beginning with the recommendation that he pay closer attention to what his wife wants or needs.

Completing column five of the chart can be discouraging unless you can consider creative ways to solve the problem. As you can see from the gift example, there is usually more than one way to get to a number better than zero. If one approach doesn't work, try something else (like, in the above example, buying the present yourself). We'll talk more about finding creative solutions to marital problems in chapter 11.

From the Web: You Need to Make It Rewarding for Both of You

If you want your husband to give you flowers and cards more often, then give him flowers and cards over and over again. *Don't* send flowers to his work. Just buy a nice floral arrangement and a card. Put the flowers in a vase on the kitchen table and set the card beside it for him to find when he notices it. And don't expect a card or flowers for every one you send. If you treat his displays of affection like you are keeping score, one of you will drop out of the race—most likely him.

When he does make even the slightest gesture of affection, even if it is as simple as telling you, "You look lovely this morning," then go overboard with your appreciation. I went for a year and a half of telling my husband I needed more affection from him, I even told him flat out that I wanted him to tell me I was beautiful. At first he didn't respond to my expectations. But one day, when he paid me an unexpected compliment, I stopped what I was doing and hugged him and kissed him and told him how much that meant to me. I began to do that every time he did something nice for me. And guess what? He pays a lot more attention to me now. I hear that I am beautiful almost every day, along with plenty of "I love you" and "You are the best thing that has ever happened to me." You need to make it rewarding for both of you.

—Jenny, 27, married five years

❧ SOME EXPECTATIONS MAY NEVER BE MET

I have always wanted to see Walt Disney World's Animal Kingdom Safari in Orlando. I would like my wife to join me. She has no interest, and she's firm about this. On this point, my hopes rank very low, no greater than a 1, and I don't have much evidence that I can change that. In this instance I might paraphrase the words of author Stephen Crane in his Civil War book *The Red Badge of Courage*: "It appears that the swift wings of my desire would shatter against the iron gates of the impossible." For some of the items in column one, there really may be very little realistic possibility of having your expectations met.

Shooting too high?

Sometimes you may underestimate your mate's capacity to meet your expectations. But you may also be overrating his or her potential, which will lead you to think that he or she just isn't trying hard enough. The fact is that your partner may be limited by physical or emotional constraints that make it impossible to do some things that you do easily. For example, a person with an autism spectrum disorder—which is characterized by an impaired ability to read interpersonal cues, body language, or tone of voice—is going to have a hard time engaging in chitchat and may not show social skills desired by the partner. The wife with a spectrum-disordered husband thinks, "He has a mouth and ears. He is no more impaired than I am. He just doesn't *want to* be social." In this case, the wife might be inclined to score the husband highly on "likelihood of attainment" based on unrealistic hopes that a medical condition can be willed or treated away.

For some people, a past trauma triggers sexual and emotional problems that can emerge years after the traumatic event. When a husband who expects a vigorous sex life sees his wife's sexual interest decline, he often assumes that the change in her sexual interest represents less interest in him, particularly if her sexual appetite was greater while they were dating. Thus, when he goes to fill in this chart, he gives her high marks on her potential, figuring either she should change her ways or he could change his ways and get a better outcome. He deserves credit for his hopefulness. But it's a mistake to think that solving this problem is simply a case of mind over matter. Helping a person recover from the emotional scars of a past trauma may require intensive therapy over quite some time.

Similarly, being unwilling to experiment with new sexual activities may seem like a simple lack of willingness on the part of a partner. But if one partner has certain sexual turn-ons that are simply off the radar map of his or her partner, it may not be reasonable to expect a high likelihood of attainment. It doesn't mean that one's partner should not experiment—you'll never know if you'll like something until you try. But, if there are moral or religious objections, if your partner is physically offended or squeamish, or if it's been tried a few times with no success, then it's time to add it to your list of "unlikely to achieve."

While we're on the subject, I strongly advise against including swinging or "adding another sexual partner" on any list of partner expectations. I have not addressed this issue in this book before now because, frankly, switching up marriage partners is just too dangerous for most marriages. I have heard it argued vociferously by pro-swinging groups that well-managed partner swapping (including setting clear rules, limiting the amount of contact with any one partner, maintaining anonymity, and so on) can be very successful. I'm skeptical. From a purely practical point of view, it breaks the marriage vows of fidelity. But beyond that, I believe it is too hard to separate out the heart from the sexual organs. People tend to feel an attraction to people they are having sex with. Perhaps that's on the basis of the surge in oxytocin that is produced during orgasm, generating a chemical effect causing two people to bond emotionally.

With these caveats in mind, give some thought to each of the expectations you have listed, and give your partner as realistic a score as you can. Here's what our sample chart looks like as we prepare to move into the last column:

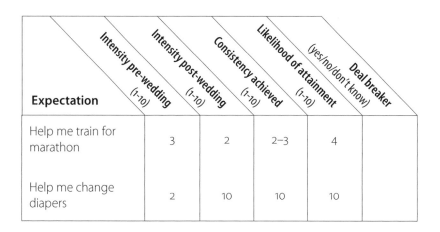

Expectation	Intensity pre-wedding (1-10)	Intensity post-wedding (1-10)	Consistency achieved (1-10)	Likelihood of attainment (1-10)	Deal breaker (yes/no/don't know)
Help me train for marathon	3	2	2–3	4	
Help me change diapers	2	10	10	10	

❧ THE BREAKING POINT

So far we have focused on the expectations you have created for your partner, both ideally—in the early days of your relationship—and as you have gotten to know him or her better. You've even considered where your mate is on the spectrum of room for improvement on the items in your list. Now it's time to think about an important question: just how essential are these issues in the grand scheme of things? Which of these expectations, if unmet, will make you decide not to stay married?

In the sixth and last column of this chart, I am asking you to take a good long look at all of the expectations you listed and ask yourself, "Is this a make-it-or-break-it issue?" In other words, "If my partner fails to fulfill this particular expectation, I will leave the marriage—legally, physically, or emotionally."

Which of the following would cause you to pack up your bags, call a lawyer, and move back into your parents' home?

- Badly made tuna sandwiches
- Arriving late for appointments
- Not helping out with triathlon training
- Not helping change the diapers

Not one of these failings would prompt most people to leave a marriage. That's not to say that these transgressions don't drive you to distraction. They simply won't cause you to divorce.

What if your partner were to do *all* of these things? Would that be a different story? Many people who decide to divorce view marital errors like water dripping on a rock: the drops of letdowns eventually cause a Grand Canyon of resentment. Although your heart may be telling you this is a good way to look at your problems, I'd like to talk to your mind for a minute: *Do not lump problems together.* Research tells us that we give five times more significance to negative interactions than we do to positive ones. It is human nature to pay more attention to difficulties in relationships than to things that go well. If you lump together all the ways your partner does not meet your expectations, you're bound to miss opportunities to see the ways he or she does. You must make an active decision to find the positive, or you will be left with the impression that the bad outweighs the good, even when the opposite is true.

I stated earlier that most people are disappointed with what they're getting in their marriage compared with when they were dating. That might seem like an argument against marriage, but really it's an argument in favor of clear perceptions. A wife who says about her husband that she feels like she has a third child is someone who pays attention to what she isn't getting from her husband. She may be overlooking that this "child" brings home a hefty salary and packs up the car and drives for cross-country trips. When's the last time your toddler brought home a paycheck or put air in the tires? If spouses focused on the many ways their mates contribute to their health and happiness, they would realize that in some ways they are getting much more than they got when they were dating.

Before you fill in the last column of this chart, think about each of the expectations you listed. Think about each one *separately from the others.* For each expectation, ask yourself: "Is this the hill I want to die on?" As you go through the list one by one, you may see that there are very few—or none—even worth considering leaving your marriage over.

In my years of counseling couples, I have found a big difference between what people believed they had to have for a successful and happy marriage and what people truly needed for marriage to thrive. But some expectations are absolutely necessary for a healthy marriage. Above all, a committed relationship must be a place where each partner can feel safe. For that reason, if domestic violence is part of the relationship, or if a partner continues with extramarital sexual partners with exposure to STDs, or if he or she is involved in substance abuse or addiction, then that behavior may present a dangerous environment for one partner (or the children) to stay in, and separation may be the only secure option. Your own safety and your family's safety is an expectation that should never be compromised.

From the Web: When You Really Think about It . . .

Marriage has peaks and valleys. Sometimes I think I have a successful marriage and other times I think it could be better. But one thing I can say when I wonder if I am truly happy is that I still love him and care about him. On a scale from one to ten, I have ten when things are going great. When things aren't going so great, it is probably around three to five. During those times, I remind myself to be more attentive, patient, and loving and soon things will be a ten again.

For me, a successful marriage is not always going to seem successful, but when you look hard enough, it really is.

—Jayne, 43, married thirteen years

❧ THE CASE FOR SETTLING

Earlier I promised I would return to a discussion of Lori Gottlieb's book *Marry Him*. I think you'll agree that her list of desires was absurdly long and mainly silly (and I didn't even include half of it). But if you look at the qualities listed, with the possible exception of height and hair volume, they are all reasonable in terms of what you might look for in someone you would choose to marry. One reason Gottlieb was single, though, was because no person exists who has all those qualities wrapped up in one. And if he had existed, he probably wouldn't be interested in her unless she was just as perfect. Which she is not, as she readily admits.

As Ms. Gottlieb learns in the course of researching her book, she has to limit what makes it on to her list of "absolutely essential." Yet, whenever she would meet with a dating consultant, she resisted taking anything off the list. As the book progresses, Ms. Gottlieb finally agrees that in the world of possible suitors, she couldn't have it all. In the end she narrows it down to three "must haves" and learns to let go of unrealistic expectations. Hence the subtitle of the book: *The Case for Settling for Mr. Good Enough.* Every married person knows what Ms. Gottlieb comes to realize: in choosing a person to marry, you have to make some compromises.

From the Web: No Such Thing as Shared Decisions

It's simple (sometimes). Assert your opinion always, but when you feel that your spouse needs to win this one, let them. Is it really that important, or do you just have control issues?

In my opinion, decisions can be arrived at with input from both people, but "decisions shared equally" can never happen. Somebody has to make the decision and see that it happens. I like to think that in my twenty-five-year marriage, the spouse who has shown the most skill in an area makes the final decision, taking into account the anxiety level of the other spouse.

❧ THIS ONE MATTERS

Now let's look again at your list of expectations for your mate. Surely it includes "Staying faithful." Almost everyone includes this one. And almost everyone says that it's an expectation worth fighting for. Yes, I agree. In contrast to so many of the expectations over the course of a relationship, this one ranks very high. To some people, nothing is more important. Many people tell themselves even before they ever choose a life partner that they would never stay if an affair happened.

You might have been one of those people. You might still be thinking of leaving. But for now, you're reading this book, so there's a chance that you'll consider keeping the marriage together.

It's okay to write "yes" in the "deal breaker" column for an item like infidelity. Writing "yes" in the final column of the chart for any of your expectations doesn't mean that, if your expectation isn't met, you have to immediately pack your bags and move out, or pack your spouse's bags and drop them by the front door. It does mean that you've narrowed your definition of what it will take to keep your relationship moving forward. And it means that these are the issues you have to discuss and work through with your mate.

Take a few minutes now to go back to the chart and complete the last, and most important, column. Here's how our sample chart looks when it's complete. Not surprisingly, neither diaper changes nor marathon training is a make-it-or-break-it issue.

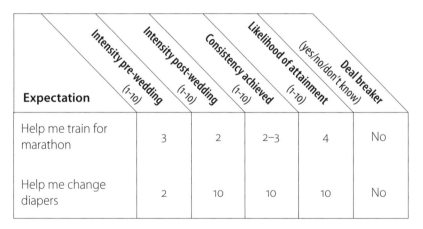

Expectation	Intensity pre-wedding (1-10)	Intensity post-wedding (1-10)	Consistency achieved (1-10)	Likelihood of attainment (1-10)	(yes/no/don't know) Deal breaker
Help me train for marathon	3	2	2–3	4	No
Help me change diapers	2	10	10	10	No

I implore you to take the time to complete your chart in writing. Recording your expectations and how you feel about them really helps. When you've completed the exercise, I hope you will take away these key points:

1 You have many expectations for your marriage and your marriage partner.

2   Many of these expectations have changed over the course of
    your marriage.

3   You may have lost hope that some of these expectations can
    be met, but perhaps there are better ways for you to help your
    partner "get it right."

4   Some of your expectations may not be based on realistic views
    of your spouse's capabilities.

5   It's better to deal with each expectation on a case-by-case basis,
    rather than lump together disappointments.

6   Pay attention to the positive contributions your partner makes,
    which can be easy to overlook.

7   Many people find that their partners come up short. But it's
    not important how many of these expectations have not been
    fulfilled. Instead, the best predictor of your marital happiness is
    your attitude about which expectations are do-or-die and your
    partner's ability to meet those expectations.

Like Anna Karenina, you may lament that your partner's ears are
too big, but, unlike her, you may come to realize that it just doesn't
matter. You have prioritized your expectations. In the next chapter I
show you how to use this information to answer a question that may
still be on your mind: Can this marriage be saved?

10

Ready to Rebuild?

THE NEXT CHAPTER DESCRIBES how to build an awesome marriage. Should you bother to read it? You may feel worn thin by the challenges that an affair brought your way. Is it worth moving forward? This chapter will help you figure out whether you're ready to read the next chapter, because when you finish reading this chapter, you will be left with one vital question: Are you ready to rebuild your marriage?

Thirty-seven-year-old Amber writes:

I got so caught up in the everyday living that I seem to have forgotten about what is really important. I was going to school full time and caring for two young children and my husband. Needless to say, I wasn't as emotionally connected to my husband as he wanted me to be, or as I wanted to be, and I wasn't communicating with him, either.

I thought everything was going okay, even though we had occasional spats, but I was sure blindsided by an affair I found out that my husband was having. Boy, was that a wake-up call. We have been married for eleven years and never once did he even bat an eye at another woman. The affair

woke me up to the fact that I was neglecting my husband and family. I wish
I could get those days back and change what happened because, even
today, I struggle with the issues the affair raised. I want to trust him because
I love him. Otherwise I wouldn't have married him.

I think this was a wake-up call in every aspect of our life, from communication to the bedroom. Counseling has been a part of our family and
probably will be for a long time. I hate knowing that he had an affair and the
lying that went with it, but it made me realize a lot of things that I needed
to learn about myself as a person, mother, wife, and friend. We are divorced
now but still live together, trying to get our relationship healthy again and
hopefully remarrying will be in the near future for us together.

If you completed the chart in the previous chapter, then you will
have faced the question of which expectations are the make-or-break
ones in your marriage and which are the ones where you might
change your viewpoint. Among those expectations, you deliberated
whether an affair spells the end of your marriage. Before an affair,
most individuals tell themselves, "I would never stay with my hus-
band/wife if I knew I had been cheated on." The reverse side of the
coin is an oath sometimes taken by the unfaithful spouse: "I would
never cheat on my spouse. If I ever found another person, I would
break up with my husband/wife before starting an affair."

Many relationships have come to a sudden halt because of the
beginning of, or discovery of, an affair. If you're the one whose
spouse cheated, you probably have wondered many times whether
you can stay married, either because of fears your mate might leave
you or because you no longer wanted to stay married to someone
who betrayed you (especially with no guarantee that it wouldn't happen in the future). If you're the one who has had an affair, there may
have been times when you thought your marriage would end either
because of your belief that there might be someone else for you, or,
having decided to end the affair, you felt your mate would never give
you another chance.

❧ CAN A MARRIAGE SURVIVE AN AFFAIR?

How many marriages are able to endure an affair and continue on successfully? Ten percent? Twenty-five percent? In chapter 3, I said that no one really knows how frequently affairs happen in marriages. For that reason, it's impossible to say how many marriages have faced infidelity and still forged ahead. However, my clinical experience and a review of the available literature make a strong case for believing that many more marriages than not stay together despite infidelity. I estimate that half or more of married couples who have experienced an affair will not divorce. That's one of the greatest secrets of surviving infidelity: that many, many people are able to do it. You just don't know who these people are, because they never told that an affair ever happened to them.

Considering how many people believe that infidelity would deal a deadly blow to their marriage, how can we understand the fact that so many couples end up staying together? It's because it's not easy to end a marriage, despite a belief that that is exactly what should be done after an affair—no questions asked. People confront a number of obstacles that complicate their instinctual impulse to place their wedding band on the night table and march out the door.

❧ REASONS TO STAY MARRIED

Nowhere else to go

Some people stay in marriage because they don't see themselves as having any other options. Financial reasons prevent them from divorcing their partner: they would lose life's basics, like a place to live, food to eat, or access to medical insurance for themselves and their children. For others, ending a marriage because of an affair might mean giving up a very comfortable lifestyle. The point is that there are many benefits to being in marriage, and some people are able to tolerate occasional dalliances if it means they won't lose the conveniences that come with the marital package. That doesn't mean they have to like it.

These worries aren't limited to one sex. Historically, most women were financially dependent on their husbands and faced poverty if they divorced. In recent years, though, many more women are the financial heavies, and their husbands rely on them for security.

Fear

Even people who are financially stable and who might sustain or even improve their lifestyle after divorce may be held back from leaving their partner by the stark reality of the big step they must take: a step into the unknown. When you think about how your entire future had been tied to that one day you shared your nuptials, then moving out of that future into a different future can be daunting. Will you be lonely? Will you be able to manage your household? What happens to your shared friends when you split up? How will your family react to your decisions?

Mackenzie was a young teacher when she married Nick, also a teacher. During the summer break from teaching, Nick went on a two-month fishing excursion with some old friends. During that time Mackenzie became closer to her summer job coworker, a divorced clinical psychologist with a cute-as-a-button son. Mackenzie and her new friend started a sexual relationship, and when Nick returned home she knew that she must end the marriage to pursue this new and exciting relationship. She had no kids, no financial burdens, not even any religious or moral guilt about the decision to end it with her husband. But she was petrified. "Nick was so angry at me; I really worried that he'd end up being hospitalized. My family had known Nick since I was in high school, and I worried that they would be disappointed in me. I kept thinking about everything that could go wrong and realized that I was going to do something there was no turning back from."

Mackenzie's divorce went through, and three years later she ended the affair with the psychologist. Today she is happily married to her second husband and has two thriving children. But she still sees her decision to leave Nick as being one of her greatest acts of bravery.

A person's decision to leave a marriage may also be affected by the risk of physical violence. Some partners choose to keep the relationship intact despite this risk. But the risks are sometimes too high and staying becomes dangerous. That's when the endangered person should get help from counselors, domestic violence shelters, or the police.

From the Web: Guardian and Protector

When I found out about my husband's affair, my emotions ranged from amused to sadness, anger, and confusion to hopelessness. To this day, I'm still thoroughly confused and stunned.

Infidelity breaks that bond between husband and wife. I saw my husband not only as a sappy soul mate, but also as my guardian and protector . . . my wingman. (I never realized I felt this way until this happened.)

Now I have trust issues, I don't even feel safe with him driving the car! Deep down, I know it was his random act of horniness that led me to feel this way. Not only am I not first in his thoughts, but my well-being is of no consequence to him, as long as he is satisfied. It cuts way deeper than a few tears and arguments. It's grief, embarrassment, abandonment, and many other things.

Shame

Another reason people hesitate to leave a marriage is shame over the affair. Journalists frequently ask me whether people get out of marriage too quickly these days. I don't hesitate to say yes. Before 1950, the divorce rate in the United States was less than 25 percent. By the early 1980s that number skyrocketed to 50 percent. I believe that our culture of "I deserve the best for myself" has led many people to focus on how their marriage disappoints them, and they rest their hopes in the dream that they'll be better off the next time around. Since I don't know Kim Kardashian, I can't say for sure whether she falls into that category. Here's what I do know: seventy-two days into marriage to Kris Humphries, her second, she released a statement: "After careful consideration, I have decided to end my marriage. . . . I had hoped this marriage was forever, but sometimes things don't work out as planned." Kim, like almost half the American population, felt it was necessary to end her marriage to look elsewhere for eternal love. In reality, divorcing one person doesn't necessarily open the way to finding the right person, since, on average, second and third marriages are less likely to work out than first marriages.

The change in society's perception of divorce, and the media attention to failed celebrity marriages, has a subtle effect on how people feel about divorce. With each report of another "failed" marriage in Hollywood (and in the neighborhood), the stigma of divorce lessens. However, many people still feel as if ending a marriage is a sign of weakness or failure. They believe others will judge them harshly for divorcing regardless of the reason. They grew up hearing, "Divorce doesn't happen in *our* family." For them, the idea of leaving a partner is anathema. They take pride in their ability to make things work out even in very trying circumstances.

For people in this situation, being confronted with infidelity does not trigger the emergency escape plan but is absorbed as an unpleasant marital task: focusing on cleaning up in the aftermath of an unfaithful spouse while the marriage marches on. Staying together because you don't feel you have an option to leave isn't necessarily a bad thing. Many long-married people who grew up "not believing" in divorce report that there were times when their shame kept them from separating, but they look back at their decades of marriage feeling glad that they stayed together to work it out. The converse is also sometimes true: individuals have endured violence, abuse, and intolerable conditions in a long marriage because they were too embarrassed to take the necessary steps to flee into safety.

Obligation

Some people want stay with their partner because they believe they have a moral, legal, or ethical obligation to do so. Their beliefs may reflect their culture—for example, some people with strong religious backgrounds see divorce as a sin. They may also grow out of individual experience. One woman I treat had a mother who had been divorced multiple times, exposing her to a parade of different men in the home. She swore that if she were ever to marry, she would make it her duty to stay "until death do us part." In some cases, this level of commitment defines the marriage and helps people find ways to heal from infidelity. However, sometimes the reverse happens: when a partner knows that his or her spouse will never leave, it presents him or her with a carte blanche for every kind of marital abuse and neglect.

A quote from Thornton Wilder's *The Skin of Our Teeth* bears repeating here because it so neatly frames the link between a sense of duty and the quality of marriage: "I didn't marry you because you were perfect. I didn't even marry you because I loved you. I married you because you gave me a promise. That promise made up for your faults. And the promise I gave you made up for mine. Two imperfect people got married and it was the promise that made the marriage. And when our children were growing up, it wasn't a house that protected them; and it wasn't our love that protected them—it was that promise." For some people the "imperfection" of their partner includes their infidelity, and their commitment to stay married is the driving force keeping them together.

Love

Another reason marriages survive infidelity: love. If only ending a relationship were as easy as saying, "I hate him/her" and filing divorce papers. People marry for a reason, and high on the list, perhaps highest in cultures where brides and grooms get to pick each other, is love. Maybe the love that brings people together is just that chemical mix called infatuation. But from meeting, to dating, to exchanging vows, to honeymooning together, to having sex, to raising children, to sharing lives together, the love that develops between two married individuals is complicated and deep. Often deeper than one betrayal can negate.

In this book I addressed the biological parts of falling in love. When I hear people say "I love him/her, I'm just not in love with him/her," I know that they are well past feeling the chemical rush of infatuation. Mature love grows over time and through shared experiences. It differs from the love you feel for your children or parents because it includes the dimensions of choice and romantic attachment. It differs from the love of a friend because friendships are optional and (presumably) nonromantic. When your relationship is going well, you hold on to your strong love as a source of guidance, strength, and consistency. When you feel enraged at your partner for his or her transgressions, this love still exists, although it often feels confusing and sometimes confining. The whole experience is even more troubling when either someone else professes love for your partner or your partner claims to love someone else.

Love is intertwined with many other experiences that empower a long-term committed relationship, like trust, reliability, empathy, and the expectation that "you have my back." Many of my clients who have been hurt by their partner's unfaithfulness struggle with trying to sort through how they can continue to love in the face of such disappointment.

When an affair occurs, some of the building blocks of mature love fall down. Love forms such a strong link from you to your spouse, what are you supposed to do? Moreover, you're not even sure what part of the marital strife is your mate's fault and what responsibilities are yours.

Consider this contribution to my Internet forum:

Honesty is the most important thing to my husband. I broke my husband's trust a long time ago by lying to him about stupid little stuff that shouldn't have mattered.

I am also a very jealous person. I thought I was over that but apparently not. When my husband and I first started dating, he had many female friends most of whom he dated in high school. I had a hard time accepting this and would accuse him of cheating. Soon I began to talk to other guys but didn't tell him about it. So my lies became bigger. I would get caught every time, and he would always give me another chance. Finally, my lying stopped. I have not lied to him at all, and I understand how important it is. I think he wants to believe that but has a hard time after all the other lies. I can accept this, and I am willing to take the time he needs for me to prove it.

We last separated about three years ago for almost a year. I wasn't lying to him; we just had a hard time getting along. I wasn't giving him what he needed and he didn't feel appreciated. I put others in front of him. During that year, we talked a lot about all our issues. I assured him that things would be different and that I have changed. He came back home and things were going much better, until he started talking to other women. Mostly I am okay with this, but two of them worry me. One is over the Internet in a game that he plays but the other is the old ex-girlfriend. He has always been very open and honest about talking to them but some of the stuff I have seen in messages hurt me. He has never given me any reason not to trust him. He has been doing little things to make me feel very loved. Even still, I started going through his e-mails and his phone to find messages and never found anything until a couple of days ago.

He is extremely angry that I went behind his back and checked his phone and e-mails and feels I'm starting my lies all over again. He said I should've come to him and asked him about it instead. I didn't think he would let me see the messages. He now will not talk to me and will not sleep in bed with me. He continues to talk to this other woman and says it's nice to talk to someone where there is no bad blood. He wants me to trust in him and believe in him and I truly want to.

I love him and want to only be with him. I want to get over this jealousy issue I have and get rid of these fears I create in my head. But how do I make him believe this?

This wife had challenged the trust of her husband early in the relationship, but more recently she sees his behavior as a challenge to her. Ultimately it is their love for each other that keeps this young couple working on their partnership. And work it is.

This story also illustrates that very difficult line between maintaining appropriate boundaries and accepting your partner for who he is (in this case, a man who has always maintained close friendships with attractive women but was open about it).

In the previous chapter, I supported Lori Gottlieb's contention, in her book on marrying Mr. Good Enough, that seeking a mate requires setting realistic sights, even being willing to "settle." People who choose to marry an imperfect individual understand this. However, even though people will settle when they choose their mate, they often seem to feel that the very act of marrying will somehow produce the qualities that were missing. Do you recall the advice sung in *Guys and Dolls?* "Marry the man today and change his ways tomorrow." If you didn't know before marriage, you know now, that people seldom change in major ways. If she drank too much before you married, she may still drink a lot. If he shopped too much before the marriage, he may still shop a lot. If he obsessed over *Star Wars*, he'll still obsess; if she cursed like a sailor, she'll still curse. If your man enjoys the company of other women, or your woman enjoys the company of other men, then that may be part of what you've chosen. You may not be in a position to change it, but you can negotiate how it should be done.

♣ PUTTING IT ALL TOGETHER

You can probably think of other reasons why people stay in marriages when they desire to leave. Counselors whose therapeutic approach is rooted in helping you seek individual happiness will say, "Ignore your fears, your shame, your sense of obligation, and the pragmatic issues; none of these things should stand in the way of your true happiness." I don't agree with that advice. I don't think these factors should be, or can be, so easily set aside. Your decision to marry was never about your individual happiness alone; it was about creating something new, and that creation would be a conduit to a different, better happiness. From climbing mountains to learning new languages, humans understand that happiness comes from completing challenges successfully; sometimes keeping a marriage together is a difficult task; leaving won't necessarily make you happier.

That may be one of the reasons why you are reading this book and not reading a stack of papers from the lawyer—because you have given thought to staying the course despite the pain of an affair.

So before we move on to the next section, take a moment to revisit these reasons, and ask yourself, how do they affect you (for example, "Fear: very afraid of being on my own")? These are meaningful financial, psychological, and cultural barriers to divorce that you should pay attention to. They will affect not only whether you decide to leave, but also how you will feel about it now and for the rest of your life.

Nowhere else to go_____

Shame_____

Fear_____

Obligation/Commitment_____

Loving feelings toward my spouse_____

Other_____

Looking at the whole picture

I believe that people survive infidelity because they eventually recognize that the unfaithful person is more complicated than the act he or she committed. I often hear the person who carried out an affair described as "a good human being," "a great father/mother," or "very attentive spouse." The one moniker that no longer applies is "faithful." But short of that, there might be a long list of good qualities.

An affair forces you to take a close look at all aspects of the relationship. Sometimes, ironically, it helps you see positives in the personality or behavior of the unfaithful spouse. Also, as Amber describes at the beginning of this chapter, an affair can help you to see areas where you yourself have fallen short. That is not to say that your shortcomings can ever justify another person's jeopardizing or leaving the marriage for an intimate relationship, but one partner's decision to commit adultery can give the other partner an opportunity to assess the contributions each has made to the problems of the marriage and what each can do to help it move forward. If you've been cheated on, and you choose not to end the relationship, you will eventually be able to make a mental list of those things about your partner and your relationship that counterbalance the affair.

I have asked you to explore your own expectations for marriage and weigh the realities and priorities that could help you decide what you really need in the relationship. As you move forward, and ultimately make an effort to choose whether you want your relationship with your spouse to continue, it will be helpful to take a close look at some of the qualities that are worth keeping in your life. Is it still worth having someone around who is a good parent? who enjoys football as much as you? who has a great sense of humor?

Obviously, most people would agree that one quality worth keeping is fidelity. I understand that your partner got it wrong this time, but not every person who cheats will forever cheat under any circumstance. If having your spouse be unfaithful once is your limit, then so be it; but for some people it's not enough in and of itself to tip the scales. What are the qualities that weigh on the positive side of the scale? Use the chart on the next page to rank some of the better qualities of your mate. For each quality, ask yourself, what's it worth? How many stars does your mate earn? There's space at the end of the chart to add other qualities that you pay attention to:

Pays attention to my needs	★ ★ ★ ★ ★
Is prompt and on time	★ ★ ★ ★ ★
Has a great sense of humor	★ ★ ★ ★ ★
Has a good relationship with my family	★ ★ ★ ★ ★
Is really talented artistically	★ ★ ★ ★ ★
Gets into the same things I do	★ ★ ★ ★ ★
Is a great parent/aunt/uncle	★ ★ ★ ★ ★
Helps to calm me when I'm upset	★ ★ ★ ★ ★
Is generous	★ ★ ★ ★ ★
Helps me solve problems/fix things	★ ★ ★ ★ ★
We have satisfying sex together	★ ★ ★ ★ ★
I feel connected when we talk about things	★ ★ ★ ★ ★
Is great to have in a real crisis	★ ★ ★ ★ ★
Provides well for me financially	★ ★ ★ ★ ★
Engages in interesting conversation	★ ★ ★ ★ ★
Is spiritually elevated	★ ★ ★ ★ ★
Cooks well or is otherwise nurturing	★ ★ ★ ★ ★
Will fight for me if I need it	★ ★ ★ ★ ★
Really knows how to relax	★ ★ ★ ★ ★
_____	★ ★ ★ ★ ★
_____	★ ★ ★ ★ ★
_____	★ ★ ★ ★ ★
_____	★ ★ ★ ★ ★
_____	★ ★ ★ ★ ★
_____	★ ★ ★ ★ ★
_____	★ ★ ★ ★ ★
_____	★ ★ ★ ★ ★

When the bad outweighs the good

It's worth taking a good look at what your partner can do right. But sometimes, no list of good can outweigh certain bads. Serial, or ongoing, infidelity is one such example. If your partner continues to return to the same unfaithful behavior repeatedly, that should be a big red flag—it should alert you that the person's flaws cannot be easily overshadowed by his or her good points. What follows is a Web-based contribution from a woman living overseas. Her story has a happy ending, but her marriage did not. As the dates indicate, the time line goes for several years.

Feb 6: I have been married for ten years. My husband had a one-night stand six years ago that resulted in a baby. I forgave him and decided to move on. It wasn't easy. The woman gave full custody of the child to my husband, and I have been raising the child as my own. But he continued to look outside the marriage. I first found letters, and it went on from there. I was always hoping deep down he would change.

Lately my husband always has his mobile phone off, and I noticed he would make trips late afternoon or night to the library or to buy milk, even though we had enough. Then I got his mobile bill at the end of last year, and there was this long list of the same number. I called it. Of course a woman answered. She told me they were only friends. I confronted him really sternly, and his only response? Silence and more silence. He doesn't even say "sorry." I am seriously thinking of leaving this time. Still I am trying to leave a window for him but that window is getting smaller and smaller.

Feb 9: I spoke to the "friend" again. She says he didn't sleep with her; he just liked how much "attention" and listening she was giving him. But I have to recognize I was letting myself go in the marriage too. It is a big eye opener to me because even though he is much at fault, there are things in me I need to change.

Feb 12: I just came back from a trip with my husband. We talked. He said that it was a stupid thing to do and he would try to change some things.

Well, first time ever I heard him talk like that! After a while I told him we could try *one* more time, only once, that is it.

At this point on the message board, 36-year-old Zach adds his contribution:

Feb 24: I don't want to be the devil's advocate here, but your husband is a cheat. And once a cheat, always a cheat. You have put up with way more in this marriage than most women would. He has cheated on you more than once, the time resulting in your stepson, the woman on the other end of the cell phone (yes they were having an affair, don't delude yourself), and the times you know nothing about.

Taking you to the beach for your romantic getaway was "damage control." He is facing the fact that you are going to leave. He is looking down the barrel of a divorce. Child support, financial strain, isolation from the kids, and he is scared. But he will cheat on you again, I can guarantee it.

Don't delay the inevitable. Get out of this toxic relationship *now*, and find someone who will be faithful to you.

And *do not* blame yourself for his atrocious behavior. It is *not* your fault he is a dog.

So, dear reader, where do you stand on the issue? Are you a believer that this husband will turn things around, or do you agree with Zach? Read on:

Feb 28: This week I thought everything was okay, except for some arguments. Then, I got to see some messages in the old phone my husband had, and found out my husband and his "friend" had no morals and were the biggest liars; they were taking me for a ride all the time.

I don't want more apologies. The relationship is toxic. That's it! I have had enough. I can't take it any longer, so sick of begging and being left alone and feeling like a potato sack in the corner. I'm moving out.

Aug 21: Although my husband kept saying he couldn't stand the situation, he wouldn't do anything about it. Now I realize I held on too long to this marriage. It has been hard some days but the support of family and friends has been huge. I am so much calmer and relaxed now.

It will take me a long time to trust someone and put the effort in another relationship in the future.

April, the following year: Well after so long, what can I say? That I am as happy as I could ever be. Not because my situation got better, but I am free! Finally got to break away from all that pain that was holding me really bad. I have lost now sixty-seven pounds and have guys asking me out every week! It's good to feel alive again, but this didn't come without a price and many months of pain as well. As much as it hurts to leave some things behind, the future gets better. My ex-hubby is not very happy, but honestly what did he expect? I had enough of his games, even to this day he is still seeing the woman I contacted before I left.

So just to let you know if some women are going through the same, don't give up! Go and live your own life instead of getting bitter with someone who is *never* gonna change.

June, two years later: Hmm, I forgot for a while I had posted something like this, and reading it back over I find it hard to believe I had such a life. I have matured. I have grown as a person and found an incredible man. He loves me so unconditionally and treats me so well, the way we all deserve. He knows all about me. I am being totally honest because this time I am not holding back on something that doesn't feel right.

Zach was right: this woman's husband was a liar who kept on lying. Such a man inflicts cruelty on someone by continuing to see other people, continuing to have illicit relationships, and continuing to lie, all while telling his wife that there is something wrong with her. While I am a strong advocate for marriage, it's hard for me to justify supporting a long-term committed relationship when one partner simply does not demonstrate the capacity to stay away from other intimate relationships. Sometimes leaving is the wise thing to do.

❧ WHAT NEXT?

If your relationship has been put on hold—if you are physically separated, if divorce proceedings have been filed, or if one or both of you have shut down communication or intimacy with each other—you have to answer this vital question: is it possible to start it back up?

I don't take it for granted that people who have been affected by infidelity want to read about improving their relationship. Many simply say, "Screw it, I'm done with this." Yet you forged ahead. You have weighed your own reasons for staying and taken a careful look at some of your mate's qualities that may make saving your relationship an effort worth making.

If at this point you feel it's time to bow out, I still applaud you for the effort. If you make the decision to divorce, I hope you find the journey as smooth as circumstances will allow, but I simply don't have good advice on how to go about doing that. Thank you for putting all the effort into getting this far in the book. The chapter that follows addresses ways of improving marriage, and you may want to consider reading it anyway, for future relationships. Good luck!

On the other hand, if you have chosen to forge ahead in the marriage it means you have weighed your own reasons for staying and taken a careful look at some of your mate's qualities that may make saving your relationship an effort worth making. Marriage is a remarkable institution, so I am always delighted when people consider finding ways to make marriage succeed. However, I also appreciate that many couples are on the fence about marital reconnection. Reading the following chapter doesn't mean you've decided for sure that you want the marriage to work, but does show a few things:

- You take your marriage seriously
- You're willing to try to find new ways to improve your marriage
- You're open to the idea that an improved marriage will reduce the chances that infidelity will happen in the future

Now comes the time to determine what "surviving infidelity" means to you. To me, it means that there is hope for your marriage.

Here are some statements to help you find out if you and your partner are ready to focus on rebuilding your marriage. You probably won't be able to agree with all of the statements, and you and your spouse may not necessarily agree with each other. But moving forward does require some basic elements that should be in place to make things move smoothly.

If I have been the victim of the affair:

1 I am able to spend more than a few minutes, sometimes more than an hour, at a time with my partner not thinking about or bringing up the affair.

2 My partner has acknowledged the role that he or she has played in the affair, and I am satisfied that he or she is accountable for what has happened.

3 I can make a conscious decision not to allow my emotions to be ruled by my hurt or anger over the affair.

4 I have developed enough trust in my partner that I feel safe to continue to move forward (even though the trust level may not be at 100 percent).

5 I acknowledge that even though the affair was not my choice, there are things I could do to improve the marriage that may reduce the chances that an affair will happen again.

If I am the one who has had an affair:

1 I have taken responsibility for the affair and recognize that the decision to have an affair was mine alone.

2 To the extent possible, I have ended all contact with the person with whom I have had an affair.

3 I have set appropriate boundaries with "attractive others" (as defined in chapter 1) to reduce the risk of having an affair again.

4 I have consistently acted in ways that will instill trust in my spouse (for instance, sharing passwords, Facebook, and cell phone data).

5 Having granted myself enough forgiveness for what I have done, I am not mired in self-contempt.

6 I appreciate that I have some unfulfilled needs for the marriage, but that I have to take some responsibility in getting those needs met.

How will you know if you are ready to save your marriage? You won't. Not for sure, anyway. Like deciding whether you're ready to tie the knot, ready to be a parent, or ready for any other life-changing event, you collect as much information as you can, weigh the pros and cons, and then take a leap of faith. So leap with me to the next chapter and learn the steps to a happy, healthy marriage.

11

Building a Better Marriage

As Amber poignantly revealed in the last chapter, affairs can wreck a marriage. But Amber also alludes to the fact that infidelity doesn't have to lead to divorce. Many couples create lasting and healthy marriages after one of them has an affair. My joy in being a marriage educator comes from teaching couples new ways to have great marriages. That's what I want for you. Are you ready to try?

❧ LET'S DANCE

After an affair—or even without an affair—some marriages crumble for unavoidable reasons. For example, when someone marries simply to get a green card and citizenship or when, as we discussed earlier, drug abuse, domestic violence, or serial adultery make the marriage unsafe or untenable. But most of my patients who decide not to continue their marriages do so because, even though they sought out marriage counseling, they refused to make the changes needed to save their marriage. Marriage can be taught, but you have to be willing to learn—and so does your partner.

Last year, my wife bought us a class in ballroom dancing for our anniversary. Even though I thought we both could dance, the one-hour lesson was a humbling experience. Yes, I knew that one dances a waltz to a one-two-three beat, and I had enjoyed many years of dancing it with my wife. But I didn't know that, as the dance begins, I must start with the left foot, plant the foot from heel to toe and, on my next series, start with a step backward from toe to heel. To waltz correctly, I was instructed to hold my right hand just beneath my wife's left shoulder blade and hold her hand in my left hand at just the perfect angle. I wasn't permitted to look down, and when I turned my wife, it had to be to my left. And for every rule I had for dancing the waltz, Susan had an equal but opposite rule. Several times Susan and I broke down in laughter as we struggled to keep it all together.

That's how to waltz. You might argue that not everyone has to waltz to the same rules, and I'd agree that you can have a lot of fun making all kinds of adjustments to the routine. But I'd also wager a bet that the world's best ballroom dancers, as varied as their routines may be, all started with the same basic rules.

There are basic rules to follow in marriage just as there are in dance. But, unlike in dance, it's possible (in my view) to narrow marriage down to one instruction. Just one. Once you master this rule you can creatively experience all kinds of wild and crazy things in marriage. But unless you know the rule and apply it consistently, you'll struggle to make your marriage work.

In this chapter I teach you that rule, and, with it, lay the groundwork for many years of marital happiness. But before going on, I want to clarify two issues:

1 As in chapter 9, the information in this chapter is not directed only to people who have suffered from an affair; it applies to

everyone who has ever been in, or is currently involved in, a committed relationship.

2   The following marital strategies are intended for the person reading them. They are about you, the things you need to do, and the changes *you* need to make. I know that your partner has issues. (Who doesn't?) But the advice in this chapter is not provided so you can say, "Aha! That's exactly what he/she is doing wrong!" Don't highlight passages for your partner to read. Highlight them so you can return to them and remind yourself.

Several years ago a reporter from the Huffington Post asked marriage experts from around the country to respond to the question, "How can couples have a happy marriage?" She wanted a one-sentence answer. Here's what I came up with: *Figure out what your spouse would like from you. Then, do more of what your spouse likes and less of what your spouse doesn't like.* Yeah, I know, it's two sentences, but it's my quote and I'm sticking to it.

Like the waltz's one-two-three beat, you'll notice that this rule has three simple parts: (1) figure out needs, (2) do more of the positive, and (3) do less of the negative. So let's start with the first part: how can you figure out what your spouse would like to make him or her happy?

❦ STEP 1: FIGURE OUT NEEDS

You would think that two people who meet, date, fall in love, choose to marry, live in the same home, and raise children together would have figured out by now what their partner needs. It ain't necessarily so. Wives lodge one complaint more than any other: "He doesn't listen." The most common lament of husbands is: "Nothing I do makes her happy."

Let me break down these complaints for you: one partner (studies show that 85 percent of the time it is a woman) believes she is asking clearly for what she wants. The other partner (usually a man) responds in a way that shows that he clearly understands what she is asking for. This ought to work out just fine. Why doesn't it? Underlying this marriage-busting dynamic is one common denominator: assumptions. Partner A says things and assumes that Partner B understands them. Partner B hears things and assumes that he or she understands them. So B snaps into action (or inaction) based on what he or she understood, and A watches in amazement as B does something way off base. Here's an example:

Ann: Do you think we should tell our daughter to take vitamins now that she's in college?

Bob (a physician): She's probably getting good enough nutrition through the college cafeteria.

Ann: How come you never support me? You treat me like my opinions don't matter.

Ann assumed she clearly communicated that she wanted her daughter to take vitamins. Bob assumed he was being asked for his medical opinion, and he gave a thoughtful answer. It's easy to see why Ann would look at conversations like these and say, "He never listens." It's also obvious why Bob would feel he could not say anything to make Ann happy. As outside observers, you and I can see that Ann posed her preference as a question rather than as a statement and that Bob responded as if she had sought his opinion. If couples can come to cross-purposes over something as simple as vitamins, imagine the difficulties they face when talking about really important things.

It's all about communicating effectively. I've touched on the topic before, so by now you know that individuals who wish to get through to each other had better become masters at communication. It's not as hard as it seems, and it starts with learning how to listen. And that means dropping assumptions.

What is communication?

Imagine the following scene in my consulting room. The woman begins: "He never communicates; I never know what's on his mind." As I look over, I see the "uncommunicative" partner shifting in his seat, shaking or nodding his head, occasionally scowling, his eyes anxiously darting about. As the session progresses, I might see that same husband reach out and hold hands with, or offer a Kleenex to, his wife. As the session draws to a close, the woman looks at me and says, "See what I mean?"

"No, I don't," I respond. "While your husband barely spoke, it was absolutely clear to me that he did plenty of communicating throughout the session. He demonstrated annoyance, anxiety, agreement, guilt, and compassion without saying a word. He didn't have to talk at all to convey information."

"Communicate" doesn't have to mean "talk." When people believe that the only worthwhile communication is an exchange of words, they miss an opportunity to appreciate all the other ways communication takes place. Being open to many different ways of communicating makes our world much richer.

Research shows that there are gender differences when it comes to communication. While it's not true for all men or all women, studies have found that women develop verbal and relational skills earlier in life. On average, compared with girls, boys seem more attracted to inanimate things than to people. Whether because of innate brain difference or because of how social pressures shape the development of their brains, men generally have a more difficult time than women translating information from the emotional part of the brain to the verbal part of the brain, so men are less likely to talk about their emotions. Many women wish their husbands would talk more about their feelings, and many men wish their wives would talk less about theirs. Put another way, talking isn't an average guy's best mode of communication.

Women often communicate in an effort to build bridges and form collaboration. A woman (like Ann, in the vitamin example above) might pose a suggestion in the form of a question, hoping to reach a consensus. Men are more likely to use words as a tool, to solve problems directly, rather than to build social bridges. As linguistic expert Deborah Tannen writes, women talk to build "rapport," and men talk to express a "report."

Very often there's a lot more communicating going on than words reveal.

Some gender-specific tips for improving communication

At a conference of the American Psychiatric Association, I gave a talk entitled "Gender-specific Neurobiological, Behavioral, and Social Influence on Human Development: Implications for Heterosexual Relationships and Couples' Therapy." When I asserted that there are fundamental differences between how men and women interact with the world, I was surprised and pleased by the overwhelming support that other psychiatrists offered. In fact, many of them described how they had held strong beliefs when they were in college and medical school that there was no difference between the sexes, only to be converted to the idea once they had children of their own. It's with that support, and the years of my own research, that I recommend some gender-specific tips for improving heterosexual communication:

Men:

- Stand still during conversation. Be present in the room, physically and mentally. Some movement will relax you, but it will make her more tense.
- Don't jump into the conversation with efforts to defend yourself or fix the problem.
- Verbally acknowledge that you are listening (say "I see," or "Really?").
- Maintain eye contact when you can. Men are biologically less likely to seek eye contact, but to your wife, locking eyes says you are listening.

- Ask your wife what she wants from you in the conversation. If she wants you to listen, listen. If she wants you to help fix something, help fix it (after you listen).

Women:

- Less is more. Be less descriptive and use fewer words. Put the main point out front, and strip away unnecessary details when you start the discussion.
- Ask for what you need. Sometimes saying, "I don't want you to solve anything, I just want you to listen" takes the pressure off both of you.
- Timing is everything. Don't approach your husband when he is distracted. You'll get 10 percent of his attention and 100 percent of his frustration.
- Think action, not talk. Men tend to be more action oriented, so use action words (such as "I want") rather than feeling words (such as "I feel").
- Move. Going on walks or riding in a car engage the action-oriented brain and can reduce his anxiety during a conversation.

Conversations that can last a lifetime

The first principle of effective communication is to *learn to listen*. When your spouse addresses you, he or she wants you to tune into his or her words. Those words have great meaning to the person who speaks them.

Think about your school days, when the teacher was asking you to interpret a passage of a book or to answer a geography question. You know the subject inside and out, and you raise your hand, hoping she'll call on you. When she calls on someone else, you put your hand down for a moment, but you hardly pay attention what your classmate says, so eager are you to have the teacher and the rest of the classroom hear your thoughts. As soon as the teacher starts to respond to the other kid's answer, your hand shoots back up. You're not listening to the teacher any more than you listened to your classmate. You want the teacher to shout out your name! When the teacher finally does call on you, you put your idea out as a thing of great importance. It is, after all, your Very Original Thought.

As you go down memory lane, think about your best teachers. They called on you when your hand went up. They seemed to understand what you were saying. They didn't make fun of you. They made you feel good that you spoke up and encouraged you to do it often. Not only did you express yourself more in this teacher's class, you learned more too.

Now think about a different kind of teacher, one who ignored your airborne hand. Think about what it was like when you finally got to express your idea in the classroom and the teacher paid no attention to you or turned to others for their opinions as if you hadn't spoken at all. Or imagine her repeating what you said in a way that was nothing like what you meant, deriding you for getting it wrong, or just plain breaking out in laughter. In any of these scenarios (and most of us have experienced them at some point in our lives), think about how, at the very moment when you feel misheard or unheard, you shut down. Your hearing and vision cloud over. You pay less attention to what is going on around you as you focus on your feelings of being ignored, misunderstood, or laughed at.

This commonplace classroom experience represents the basic mechanism of every talk that you and your partner have. On rare occasions a conversation occurs just to pass time, with neither one caring if the other is paying attention. But usually when one of you speaks, it's like you're the student in the classroom. You feel you are about to share something of vital importance. You block out what is going on until you get a chance to be heard, and then, once you talk, you wait for acknowledgment.

And your partner feels exactly the same way.

Once you realize this, you can change how you have conversations. When your partner speaks because he or she wants to launch an important idea, you are like the teacher. If you interrupt, put forward your own ideas, laugh, or misunderstand, your partner will withdraw from the conversation. When it comes time for you to state your point of view, there is almost no chance you will be heard. You can see how a conversation like this will end in frustration for everyone.

However, if, like the good teacher, you act as if everything your partner says merits your attention and appreciation, he or she will feel heard. Once that happens, your partner will also pay more attention to you. He or she will feel more comfortable with you, and his or her defenses will be diminished. Let's make sure you know how to be the kind of listener who makes people feel heard.

From the Web: Have Compassion for the Other Person's Perspective

If you can just stop for a minute and get yourself into compassionate mode, the results will surprise you. You don't have to agree or even understand the other person's perspective and vice versa, but if you just have compassion for his perspective, resolution can be reached much, much faster. Naturally, he will notice the change, which will lead to changes for both of you.

—Kaleen, 42, two years into her second marriage

Listening lessons

Some people are natural-born listeners, maybe because they don't have a whole lot to say. But you don't have to be born that way; you can become an excellent listener by consistently applying some basic skills. Like properly dancing a waltz requires paying attention to each step of the process, successful listening means applying all the strategies below all (or almost all) of the time. Even the ones that seem to be common sense. Research tells us that unless you get it right five times more often than you get it wrong, your mate will walk around with the impression that you're getting it wrong.

Perhaps the most important lesson is: Make your partner feel understood. Before you respond, are you doing your best to let your partner know that you understand what he or she is saying? Start by verifying that the message delivered was the message received. Ask questions and restate what it is that you thought you heard. This skill is called *reflective listening*.

Several times in this book I have discussed the merits of reflective listening. At its core, this kind of listening involves dialoguing in a specific format in which one partner speaks and the other person's only job is to listen and then to make sure that all of the speaker's words are comprehended. This kind of dialogue is best done when both partners know how to do it, but it can be done when only one partner knows the technique. Here's a breakdown of the steps involved:

Partner 1: States a concern

Partner 2: Echoes back the concern, seeking accuracy. Usually this begins with:

- I think I hear you saying . . . ,
- If I hear you correctly, you are saying . . . , or
- Let me see if I understand you . . . ,

and follows with a rephrasing of your partner's concern.

Partner 1: Either

- confirms and expands, or
- corrects misunderstanding

It might look like this exchange between husband and wife:

> He: I was upset when you were on the phone with your mother when I got home from work.
>
> She: If I hear you correctly, you are saying that you get upset when you find me on the phone when you get home at night. Is that right?
>
> He: Yes, that's right. I feel ignored when I walk in the door and you're talking to your mother.
>
> She: It sounds like you are saying that you feel ignored.
>
> He: I do. Maybe it's selfish of me, I don't know, but that's how I feel.

People worry that dialoguing like this will sound artificial. Yet this very affirmative method of communicating powerfully gives the speaker a real sense of being heard. That person becomes a better listener in turn.

Fine-tuning your listening skills

When you try reflective listening for the first time, keep in mind your objectives. You are working together to come up with a solution to a perceived problem. By adjusting your approach and your attitude, you'll have many fruitful conversations. Here are five lessons in how to fine-tune your listening skills.

Lesson 1: Listen to learn

This is a difficult time in your marriage. Sitting and talking with your partner is a big step. As the dialogue begins, remind yourself that your objective is not to attack your partner but to gain information that will help you to understand and to enable him or her to continue to share with you and not shut down.

You may want to shout out disagreement to some of the things you hear. When you do this, you shut down the conversation. For example, suppose the dialogue above went like this:

> He: I was upset when you were on the phone with your mother when I got home from work.
>
> She: Well, if you would be respectful enough to call and give me some idea when you were getting home, maybe I'd be off the phone.

The husband's needs get lost, and the discussion gets shifted to labeling *his* behavior as a problem. It's not likely that this couple will feel good about this conversation if it continues like this.

When you have a dialogue about infidelity, the same principles apply.

Suppose your wife tells you she cheated on you because she found out you received e-mails from your ex-girlfriend. You may be tempted to clarify—then and there—that you did not solicit the e-mails. But don't. Instead, listen to how your wife tells it from her point of view so you can see it the way she saw it. Respond by saying, "I hear you saying you were upset because I was getting e-mails from Marilyn." You'll have your chance to clarify later on, but if you try to correct her interpretation of events now, you'll end up getting bogged down in the details of your ex-girlfriend's e-mails, and you'll never move on to talk about your wife and her issues. If she doesn't get heard, then she'll never be able to hear you.

From the Web: "Best friends, no matter what"

The ability to work through differences comes from two individuals in a relationship deciding that they will be committed to being the best friends they can be, no matter what. This means being honest, talking about what bugs you, talking about what makes you happy and doing it on a regular basis.

Unhappiness exists to notify individuals that they could be doing more in various other areas of their lives. A couple who suddenly finds that they are unhappy immediately must ask themselves: Are we communicating to the best of our ability? Do we care about our partner's feelings enough to ask that question? If not, can I really say that I am truly being my partner's friend?

—Dave, 25, married one year

Lesson 2: Give yourself breathing room

As we discussed in earlier chapters, there is much you want to know, and you have every right to hear the details. But it's hard to be on the receiving end of such devastating information without feeling your blood boil. If hearing your spouse disclose things makes you begin to feel out of control, don't let emotional overload get in the way of effective communication. Studies show that when you get flooded with emotions, rational thought is almost impossible.

You have permission to take a break, but you must do so without blaming your partner. You want to say, "I can't be expected to sit here and listen to your lame excuse about why you spent your evening with that tramp instead of coming to the family Christmas party!" Rather, it's better to say, "I'm on emotional overload here. I appreciate your telling me all this, but I need to take a break to get my head together before I hear more."

Lesson 3: Recognize and respect communication differences

Remember what linguistic expert Deborah Tannen says: on average, men communicate to establish power and women communicate to build alliances. Women shouldn't take it personally when men talk excitedly (that doesn't mean they are on attack), and men shouldn't dismiss their wife's perspective just because it's not as direct as they'd like (she still wants you to understand her main point). If you misinterpret these cues, you may misperceive your partner's style as disrespect.

Lesson 4: Acknowledge and agree whenever your mate makes good points

Early in my training as a therapist, I was exposed to a key principle of marriage survival: You can either fight to be right or fight to be married. Many times you will have different opinions, but at every opportunity you should look for areas of agreement. My wife and I have a long-standing tradition. Whenever she tells me, "You're right," I ask, "Would you repeat that?" When I tell her she's right, she makes the same request of me. There's a method behind our madness. By asking for repetition, I let her know that those words mean a lot to me. I also get to hear it twice. I reinforce her for saying I'm right, and vice versa. It's true of all creatures (even whales, as we'll see later on): we do more of the things we receive reinforcement for doing. My wife and I make sure to let each other know regularly either of us has a made meaningful contribution to the conversation (for example, "That's a good point!"). It keeps the conversation moving forward.

What if you have one of those partners who *always* has to be right? You know the joke: "I always dreamed of marrying Mr. Right, I just didn't know his first name was 'Always.'" By being on alert for when the other person acknowledges you, even for small things, you will recognize that, from time to time, you *do* get *some* credit.

Lesson 5: Think before reacting

Once your partner feels understood, take some time to think things through. Is this a really important issue for you or is it one that won't make a big difference in the long run? Everyone can think of examples of getting in a big marital tiff and then not remembering why you were so mad at each other. By taking a step back and putting things in perspective, you have a chance to let an argument go even before it begins.

What's your love currency?

Being a good listener is a vital relationship skill, but another part of communication involves learning how to make sure you convey messages as well as you receive them. You would think that when you express your needs to your loved one, he or she would hear you exactly as you intended to be heard.

When it comes to getting through to a spouse, many people miss the mark because they assume that their partner understands their deeds and words the same way they do. But one person's act of kindness can be totally missed, even seen as a negative, by a partner. Demonstrating love and affection only works when one partner does so in a way that has meaning to his or her mate. The right way of giving requires finding the right "love currency." In most U.S. workplaces, the currency for appreciation is dollars. In some cultures, people use seashells as a form of money. But if I live in the United States, and week after week I paid my assistant a handful of seashells, no matter how big my smile and thanks were, my assistant would quit. Seashells have no value to her, even though they might have great value to some people.

Relationships also have currency, but the form of currency is not the same for everyone. The problem with most relationships is that one partner does not realize what currency the other partner values. No matter how highly you prize something, if it has no value to your partner, it will not be appreciated. If you treasure a clean car, and you wax and shine your wife's new Accord, she won't be impressed if she doesn't care about such things. If you love dance and bring home tickets to the Bolshoi Ballet, your partner won't feel loved by the act. Why not? Because he couldn't care less about ballet.

Leah and Max, parents of three, were a couple I treated. They perfectly demonstrate the importance of finding the proper love currency. Leah, a teacher, had on many occasions bought thoughtful and loving gifts for Max, a law professor. Leah loved presents. For Leah, giving gifts was a way of showing love. Max, in contrast, abhorred gifts. He felt that if someone bought something for him, it placed a burden on him to act as if he liked it. The pressure of showing the right response made him anxious. He also explained: "Exchanging gifts is absurd. How could anyone know what I want better than me? When I get a present, I end up being stuck with a shirt, or tie, or socks that I didn't even want, bought with money we don't have. Why am I supposed to be thankful?" Although Leah gave in love, Max became overtly outraged when he got gifts. Leah was using a love currency that Max didn't use, and neither of them was happy with the results. If you don't know your partner's currency, you'll end up feeling frustrated and unappreciated, with a spouse who feels unloved. After a few weeks, months, or years of this, relationships approach their breaking points.

Different individuals place different value on different currencies. Some people value sex as a way of bonding. Others appreciate affectionate words as the greatest act of love. I often refer couples to Gary Chapman's popular book *The Five Love Languages*, in which he defines specific love currencies—which he calls "languages"—that seem to be universally shared in all cultures:

1 Acts of service (doing things such as laundry or mowing the lawn)

2 Words of affirmation (making comments like "You look beautiful" or "You worked really hard on the project")

3 Quality time (spending time together on walks, seeing movies, fishing, and the like)

4 Physical touch (holding hands, performing massage, cuddling, sex)

5 Gifts (giving items such as music CDs, jewelry, flowers, cards)

By assigning these "love languages" to five separate categories, Dr. Chapman challenges his readers to think about what category best fits their partner. Would your wife prefer a trip to Cape Cod for the day (quality time) or a set of pearl earrings (gifts)? Would your husband prefer you to give him a loving squeeze (touch) or to tell him how great you think he is (words)? Would she rather have you to do a load of laundry (acts) or take her out to dinner (quality time)? You get the idea.

Most people's immediate response to these options would be to say, "All of the above." So, how about a trip to the Cape during which you hug each other and rave about each other's fine qualities while eating at a restaurant where you get a new set of earrings, after which you return home and the hubby runs a load of laundry? That will work just fine, wouldn't you say? The reason this sounds appealing is because most people would like everything on that list (except, for instance, Max, who hates gifts). But not everyone likes them in the same order. And that's where learning the right love language, and speaking or doing it regularly in your relationship, comes into play.

❧ STEP 2: DO MORE OF WHAT YOUR SPOUSE WANTS

Consider the following scenarios: The wife who doesn't give a hoot about automobiles spends the day waxing her husband's car. The husband who doesn't like the ballet purchases two tickets for the Alvin Ailey Dance Company and accompanies his wife. Max goes out and buys a gift for Leah. These are all examples of spouses figuring out what their partners love and doing that very thing for them—even though it has no meaning for the person doing it. In each of these scenarios, the partner figures out the love currency and then pays in it.

Pay up!

If you can discover your partner's preferred love language, you can begin to give him what he or she is seeking in the currency that is meaningful. When I talk about "paying" your partner, I don't mean handing over greenbacks after she changes the motor oil or he cooks a nice meal. I am suggesting you say "I love you" and "I appreciate you" in ways that are meaningful to your partner. Happily married couples regularly let their partners know that their very existence is worthy of celebration and reward.

You heard me right. I'm advising that husbands and wives should celebrate their partners and make them feel good just because breath is still coming out of their nostrils. Many of my patients stop me midsentence when I get to this point. Either they'll point out that their partner doesn't make them feel special and therefore why should they? Or they'll say their partner has done nothing to deserve praise. Or they'll say they feel a disconnect or anger toward their partner and the *Mister Rogers' Neighborhood* overtures don't feel right. Many people mistakenly believe that praise should be withheld unless their partner achieves and maintains a certain standard of excellence.

So let me ask you: do you praise your kids? How hard do they have to work to earn an attaboy? Most parents don't insist that their child score 100 percent on every exam, sing the loudest and sweetest in the chorus, or score a run every time they are at bat. On the contrary, most parents know that when they feed children a steady diet of positive feedback for good (not perfect) acts, the children's confidence grows. Not surprisingly, these kids tend to end up feeling good about themselves, and they think highly of their parents. Some kids thrive on words of praise, some love a hug, and some expect a new video game when they get things right. Good moms and dads learn to home in on the kind of feedback, or currency, that means something to their kids and pile it on at appropriate times.

We also recognize the power of encouragement at the workplace or among friends. Yet, when it comes to our life partners, many people still hold back. I'm reminded of the book *What Shamu Taught Me about Life, Love, and Marriage,* in which journalist and author Amy Sutherland discusses a revelation she made while on assignment at Sea World. Killer whales, she reported, don't flip and spin naturally. They require constant molding of behavior by getting fish every instant they move in the right direction. Over time they do exactly what the trainers want them to do and get rewarded every step of the way. Sutherland realized that if amazing things can happen between trainers and whales, amazing things can also happen between wives and husbands. She concluded (and I agree) that improving marriage requires no criticism, anger, or punishment. It simply means throwing a meaningful reward to your mate. Your mate may not get things perfect, but a well-placed word or act of encouragement has a great chance of improving your relationship.

A fish story

One couple I worked with, Stanley and Yvonne, came to see me because of Yvonne's unhappiness with Stanley and his feeling that he could not meet her needs. For Stanley, feeling appreciated was his primary love currency. I tried to help Yvonne learn to reward him in a meaningful way using his desire for affirmation. I proposed, based on the *Shamu* book, that she buy a package of Swedish fish and "throw" Stan a fish every time she notices him do something right, while at the same time pointing out his accomplishment. She claimed the plan was doomed to fail because, in her words, "He doesn't do anything right." I've heard these objections before, and I was prepared. "Look down at his feet," I requested of Yvonne, "Do you see his shoes? Does he have each one on the correct foot?" She got my point and laughed. I instructed her that any, and I mean *any*, signs of competence should be rewarded. Even if it's as simple as putting his shoes on the proper feet.

When the couple came back two weeks later, she revealed that she had given Stanley exactly one fish, the day after our meeting. She had not given out any others since then. Despite spending half the session sorting through all the things that Stanley had been doing right (he was holding down a full-time job, helping to take the children to school, arriving home on time every night, living a substance-free life, not gambling, not fighting or arguing with her, not having an affair—and he continued to figure out which feet his shoes went on), she refused to acknowledge any positives on his part. She held to the party line that he failed at everything he tried. Imagine Stanley's frustration in the relationship. Being in a marriage deprived of your love currency is like being in the desert without water. It's deadly.

Spring thaw

Now here's a story told to me by one of my readers, Madison, who fought her inner critic and found ways to reinforce her husband, who clearly places high value on acts of service:

I am a night owl and Mark is an early bird. For many years he has wanted me to get up and fix his breakfast for him, and it has been hit and miss. When I would apologize for it he would say, "I'm used to it." But I decided to make a change. This morning I got up and made French toast and eggs, and we sat and talked even shared a few fun jokes back and forth.

Even though I was aching tired I was upbeat and happy for him. For dinner I made him baked chicken and potatoes, and as we speak I have cinnamon rolls in the oven.

Somehow we got to talking about the bills and who pays them and I said I hated doing them (it slipped), and right away he said, "But I work all day," so I got up from my chair, went over to him and said, "Yes, you do, and I love you for being such a hard worker for our family. I love you for it, you are my hero."

Here's the wild thing. We live in the country, and we ran out of wood early this spring, and Mark knows I *love* my wood heat, but earlier that month he said, "There is no more wood." Well, he went out the back door a few minutes ago in search of wood! And I know it is all because of what I did. I do know that he just wants me to take care of him and he wants to be my hero and acknowledged for what he does.

You carry in your pocket an ample supply of what your partner needs to feel special. You can choose to be like Yvonne and withhold it, or you can choose to be like Madison and dole it out in spades. Which approach will make your relationship better?

Spicing things up

Think about when you and your partner were first dating. Do you remember how you felt after the first date, when you couldn't wait to have another date? Your partner wants to get some of those feelings back. And so do you. Increasing the positive energy and excitement in your relationship is a marriage booster.

By turning your knowledge of brain chemistry to your advantage, you can bring back that sense of excitement. The two neurochemicals discussed in chapter 4, norepinephrine and dopamine, increase attention and elevate energy levels. These neurochemicals don't emerge only during infatuation, however; they are part of our body's adaptation to all kinds of stimuli in the environment. Marriage can be so very "day in, day out"—in fact, it can be downright boring. Boring can be good for a little while, especially if you are rebounding from the disrupting effects of an affair, but people feel most alive when they are challenged and excited by things in their environment. Moreover, partners become more interested in each other if they feel a spark of electricity between them.

Researchers at State University of New York at Stony Brook conducted a study in which he split married couples into two groups. They asked one group to simply walk back and forth across a room. When they interviewed these couples after this exercise, the couples felt fine, but their relationship hadn't changed at all. They gave the second group a different task. These couples were also instructed to go back and forth across a room, but to do it on all fours, with their arms and legs bound to their partner's while pushing a ball. Couples in this group said they felt emotionally closer to their partners after the challenge than they had before the challenge. The researchers concluded that excitement and cooperative effort brings people closer together. Studies like this suggest that dopamine is triggered by novel events and that noradrenaline rises with physical and mental activities.

Date night on steroids

How many times have you heard marriage experts or therapists advise couples to have a date night once a week? Okay, I'll join the chorus. But when I give the advice, I don't just recommend going to the same old familiar joint week after week so you can talk about the children or the home maintenance. I tell couples to change things up every week, try new restaurants, and order new foods. One of my clients arranged to take his wife to a cooking class/dinner at a local restaurant. After the chef taught the class how to prepare four courses, the restaurant served all the students an elegant dinner.

Add new stimuli to the marriage to help sustain your interest in each other. Think about all the possibilities:

- *Go camping together.* A new environment increases our sense of connectedness, particularly because new challenges increase the levels of the neurotransmitter dopamine. Camping tends to require shared effort but also tends to emphasize the skills and abilities that each brings to the experience.

- *Cook a meal together.* This activity focuses on cooperation and communication and has the added benefit of creating a finished product that both of you can enjoy. The smells of cooking increase your sensory experience, and the movement, combined with the heat from the kitchen, can raise your level of excitement.
- *Learn a new skill together.* Taking classes can be a fun way of connecting and learning things about each other that you didn't know before. It helps each of you to appreciate the other's abilities and neutralizes the differences between you, since you're both learning something new.
- *Create art together.* Paint, sculpt, or even color. You are integrating silence, thought, creativity, and mutuality into your daily routine.
- *Make a movie together.* It's relatively easy in these days of digital cameras and cell phone videos to create movies and post them online. While making even a short film can be a lengthy process, working together on writing, directing, and acting gives you and your spouse a chance to produce a product that you can share with the rest of the world.

From the Web: "Remember how you felt when it started"

If I could give advice to newlyweds, it would be to write down how you feel right now, the anticipation, the joy, and the passion. Keep a journal of the love and wonderment. Focus on your admiration of his wonderful qualities and the respect you have for him. Every day as you wake up, look over at the terrific guy you are married to and remind yourself of his strengths. Every evening write down a few sentences describing the funny, joyful, silly, romantic moments that you shared.

When you hit rough spots in the future, and you will—we all do—go someplace and privately read those words and let yourself feel again those feelings of joy. Look inside yourself, think about the present rough spot, and then ask yourself, "What can I do to make our situation better?" Take responsibility to move forward to a new and better place together. Marriage is a team effort. You try to ease his burdens and he will try to ease your burdens.

Most important of all, have fun. Vacuum in your underwear, eat dinner off each other's stomachs, play strip anything.

          —Pamela, 51, ten years into her second marriage

Together apart

For years, marriage experts were pushing for couples to spend more and more time with each other as a way to increase their bond. However, newer research into marital relationships led scientists to a contradictory discovery: too much time together can reduce "couple attraction." It makes sense to me, since time apart from your mate often increases your feelings of appreciation for him or her. When you are stuck on the tarmac for three hours waiting for mechanics to clear your plane to take off, it's your wife or husband that you think to call. If you can't reach him or her, that only reinforces your desire to connect. Esther Perel, author of *Mating in Captivity: Unlocking Erotic Intelligence,* reminds us that when you arrive at a party and see your spouse across the room comfortably chatting and laughing with other people, you have an increased interest and passion for him or her.

People who have been affected by affairs also understand this phenomenon. Many unfaithful spouses describe a surge in desire to be with their spouse as soon as they began a sexual relationship with their affair mate, and spouses who have been cheated on will sometimes have heightened sexual desires for the cheating mate. That's because attraction is accelerated when you drift apart. It also helps explain why many couples who get back together after an affair have a temporary boost in the frequency of sexual activity.

Stirring up an attraction

You can improve your marital attraction by purposefully putting some space between you and your spouse from time to time. In other parts of the book, I talk about the kinds of space that are not healthy, such as flirting with attractive persons or excluding your partner from your communications with others. Positive space would include things like one of you going out with your friends (who are of the sex you are *not* attracted to) or going on a mini-vacation with your family members without your partner. You can even set the stage to increase your sense of attraction by playing certain seduction games, such as agreeing to have one of you sit at a bar or club and have the other one try their pick-up skills. The cast of the popular TV comedy *Modern Family* plays this out masterfully when actors portraying the Dunfees, married parents of three teens, pretend to meet at a bar. In this scene the husband, Phil, wears a "MY NAME IS CLIVE" sticker, pretending to be an out of town guest at a convention as he tries to seduce his wife, whom he treats like an intriguing vixen. He wins her over, of course, and demonstrates that a mundane marriage can be exciting when you temporarily put some space between you and let the energy sizzle.

Sex matters

Marriages need sex

Sexual intimacy is an essential part of healthy romantic relationships. My research found that about 75 percent of men describe themselves as having a higher sex drive than their wives. In about 25 percent of marriages, a woman will have a higher sex drive. In either case, when one partner is in the position of wanting something from the other, and the other holds the key, it can stir up power struggles.

An example: A young man I treated was dating a young mother who had been through a messy divorce with her first husband. She became pregnant with my patient's child, and they decided to marry. After the birth of her second child, the wife concluded that she was excessively fertile, and she refused to have any vaginal intercourse with her husband. He would plead in frustration, but he couldn't make her have vaginal sex. The marriage ended a few years later, and another messy divorce ensued. I'm not saying the lack of sex caused the divorce, but I believe one reason this couple dissolved their relationship was that they stopped having sex.

Couples disconnect from each other emotionally if they don't engage sexually, if at least one of them desires sex. Because you are vulnerable and exposed during lovemaking, the act instills trust and produces an aura of safety with your partner. Physical touch itself reduces stress and lowers blood pressure. For people who are not able to verbalize feelings very well, sex is a powerful way of communicating feelings of love. And when couples engage in sex that includes orgasm, orgasm raises the levels of oxytocin (the bonding hormone). This can increase the intensity of the bonding between you and your spouse.

From a practical point of view, sex is an implied expectation of marriage. Propose the following hypothetical to any young man (and quite a few young women): if you had a chance to marry the person of your dreams but will never be permitted to have sex, would you tie the knot? Most would turn down the offer because, for most people, the person of their dreams is (among other things) the person they fantasize about sleeping with.

From the Web: Sex and Pregnancy

I am currently pregnant, and just the pregnancy has changed our relationship considerably. My husband and I rarely have sex anymore. I can't figure out why. It makes me feel that he is unhappy with me. He says it's just the fact that there is a baby inside me that has lowered his sex drive. I think that has put a strain on our marriage. I need to feel wanted and that just isn't happening right now.

—Jessica, 26, married two years

Saying yes to sex

When I talk to couples about connecting through sexual intimacy, I sometimes hear the objection (from the partner with lower sexual desire) that sex is fine if both partners want it. However, they point out, when one partner feels exhausted, unattractive, or preoccupied, that person is justified in putting the kibosh on sex for the night. I agree. Everyone should have the freedom to say no to sex. But if night after night one partner cannot summon the constellation of circumstances to desire sex, his or her individual needs must be weighed against the needs of the couple. I think you see where I'm going here: the low sex drive person should have sex anyway. Even if she or he doesn't feel like it.

There are gender differences to consider here. Admittedly, it is difficult for men to get an erection if they lack interest. Most women can successfully have vaginal intercourse even when they don't have the desire for sex. Studies show that women often don't realize when they are aroused and may start vaginal lubrication even before they are aware. Moreover, the belief that women must first experience desire before they can enjoy sex has been disproven. Often, just starting some foreplay with an attractive mate produces an increase in desire. As one of my patients told me, "I didn't think I was interested in lovemaking, but once I got into it, I *really* got into it." She also reminded me that as a bonus to enjoying sex, the days that followed found a marked reduction in her husband's—and her—stress levels.

Can I have sex after knowing my partner has been with another partner?

Recommending a healthy and active sexual relationship for couples with typical marital issues is fine, but is it reasonable to ask that of couples who have struggled through an affair? I see many individuals who do not feel ready to get back under the covers with their partner. Some concerns of the person cheated on include:

- My partner may have contracted an STD, and I don't want to risk exposure.
- Exposing my body and having sex makes me feel too vulnerable to future hurts if it happens again.
- I'm afraid of my own sexual desires and worry that needing my partner will take away my sense of control.
- When my partner is with me, I imagine he or she is comparing it to sex with the other person and that makes me feel ashamed and angry.

Some concerns of the partner who had an affair might be:

- What if I don't perform well sexually? My partner will assume it's because I've lost interest, when the real problem is that I'm nervous.
- I worry that when I am with my wife/husband, I will begin to think of the other person.
- If my spouse doesn't satisfy me the way my affair mate did, I may never be happy with this marriage.

Many couples who reunite after an affair have sex with each other with wild abandon. Others take their time getting comfortable with each other again, moving slowly through courting rituals—hand holding, kissing, petting—as if they were virgins. But at some time or another most couples have to confront these concerns. Just as each couple plans a wedding based on their own unique couple style, joining together sexually is going to look different for every couple. Here's one simple solution: talk. If you've moved far enough along in the relationship to try to return to the home base of marriage, you're far enough along to start to talk about sex. If you have fears about your vulnerability or performance, share them with your partner. (Remember, partner: when you hear these fears, seek first to understand them before you rush in with reassurance or a solution.) When you give each other a chance to bring concerns out in the open they lose their power and their mystery and you find relief.

Except for one thing. If you've had a sexual affair, and your partner has concerns about sexually transmitted diseases, then your job goes beyond being an active listener. Before the two of you resume sex, you should consult with your physician to take adequate steps to test for and prevent the transmission of disease. Even if your partner does not express concerns, that still should be part of your reconciliation plan.

Will you have a great sex life once you have healed from the affair? I am reminded of the classic joke:

Patient: Doctor, will I be able to play the violin after my surgery?

Doctor: Yes, of course you will.

Patient: Oh, good, because I could never play it before!

Here's the hard truth: if you weren't sexual virtuosos before, it's unlikely that you'll make beautiful music together the first time you're back together in bed. But allow me to extend this classic joke to an unfunny but inspirational conclusion:

And so at that very moment the patient recovered from surgery, she committed herself to learning the violin, and now she plays in the philharmonic.

Corny, I know. But here's the point: You may have problems in many parts of your sexual relationship. But you can meet together in the bedroom and begin a process of constructing an extraordinary sex life. It takes time, talk, and trust, but if you devote yourself to bonding more closely, the bonds of your sex life and your entire relationship will be stronger.

✤ STEP 3: DO LESS OF WHAT YOUR PARTNER DOESN'T LIKE

I don't need to write a chapter about what not to do in a relationship, because your partner can do that for you. Almost all of us know what upsets our mate because, at some time or another, he or she has told us about it. What pushes your mate's buttons? How does your behavior or habits push those buttons and harm the relationship?

A friend of mine from college often laments that his wife complains because he leaves the toilet seat up. Like many men, my friend doesn't realize is how distressing it is to sit on a toilet in the middle of the night if the seat is up. But this isn't the important point. What matters is that my friend's wife is complaining and, unless putting down the toilet seat represents some hardship for him, he ought to just do it.

If your partner has concerns about excessive use of alcohol, drug use, smoking, gambling, or pornography, I urge you to pay attention. Studies show that marriage helps protect people against a host of substance abuse and medical-related problems, probably because of the positive influence of a spouse on decision making.

Another source of couple complaints is money. If a couple is having real financial trouble, and one person continues to spend without paying attention to the warnings and pleas of the other, you know this will have a negative effect on the marriage. Sticking to the mantra of "do less of what your partner doesn't like," the free-spending spouse needs to change his or her ways.

Other common areas of complaint include childcare, housework, and in-laws. In all these areas, paying attention to your partner's needs may go a long way toward improving your marriage.

Easy for me to say

The recommendation to do less of what your partner doesn't like is based on two not-always-valid assumptions. One, that what your partner wants you to stop doing is simple enough to stop doing, and two, that your partner's desire for you to cease and desist is valid and humane.

On the one hand, some things are hard to stop doing—like smoking cigarettes or overeating. Changing these habits may involve getting professional help or even taking medication, but consider that your partner's wishes for you to change are quite valid. On the other hand, some wishes can be unreasonable. For example, some spouses are annoyed at their partner for the "habit" of staying at work until late into the evening, but if the partner just landed a first job out of college as a stock analyst in a Fortune 500 company, it's not the partner's fault that the company expects him or her to stay on through the evening. On the flip side, if the partner owns the firm and already has a very healthy bank account, then the spouse's desires are valid.

Is calling your mother every day a "habit," and is it fair for one partner to ask another not to do it? Unless your mother incessantly puts down your mate and insists thatyou get a divorce, in most cases it is not reasonable to ask one person to give up a meaningful and positive ritual. However, you might honor a request that goes, "Please don't spend time on the phone with your mother when I'm at home with you." You may not like that request, but you can follow it without undue hardship.

What if demands aren't reasonable?

It's not easy to walk the fine line between what bothers your mate and what you feel you want, or need, to do to be you. Here's a contribution to my website forum that highlights how stringent the demands of a spouse may be. The posting comes from Jack, who is in his second marriage. Jack's new wife couldn't wait until Jack's youngest child finished college so she and Jack could have nothing more to do with his first wife (now remarried). However, in Dickensian fashion, his daughter ended up marrying her stepfather's son. Now family ties bind them more closely than ever, and Jack's new wife is worried she'll never get rid of the ex-wife's influence. She is even further dismayed because she has not been able to get pregnant, and Jack's daughter is pregnant. Jack writes:

I'm not sure if you can help me, but I'm getting pretty desperate. For the most part I've felt like my wife and I had a pretty good marriage. Most of the time we get along very well and are very happy together, but my wife has always had a big problem dealing with the fact that I have been married previously.

A week ago my daughter texted me to let me know that she had had her ultrasound and all was well. I called her to let her know I was glad. My wife found out I had called her and had been talking about the baby. She flipped out. She told me I was not allowed to talk to my daughter about her baby or the pregnancy. She told me that I would not be allowed to have any contact with my grandchildren, that they were not related to us and that I was to have nothing to do with them. I had to call my daughter up and tell her that I couldn't talk to her about her pregnancy. My wife told me that I would not be allowed to go to my son's Eagle Scout court of honor this Sunday because my ex-wife and my daughter will be there. I have refused to miss this important occasion in my son's life, but she insists I will not be going.

This cannot continue. We are at the breaking point. I don't know what to do. I'm sure I have not handled things perfectly well when she has acted this way, but it was because I did not know how to react. I'm afraid to call my daughter ever. I'm afraid of setting her off and seeing her become another person—cruel and hateful, saying terrible things about my children. I can't completely cut off my daughter. I feel my wife is being unfair and irrational. I don't know what to do. Just by writing this to you I could get into big trouble if she sees it.

If Jack were to take my advice to "do less of what your partner doesn't like," he would be sacrificing his relationship to his children and his grandchildren, a connection that obviously (and rightfully) means the world to him. Therefore, Jack ought not to accept his wife's wishes, as they go against deeply held, reasonable beliefs. He will sacrifice stability in his household if he still sees his family, but he has every right, even a duty, to forge ahead. There does come a time where one partner asks for unreasonable sacrifices from the other, and standing your ground is part of maintaining your individual identity in the union.

How do you know who is right when it comes to differences of opinion on matters of the definition of what's reasonable, moral, safe, equitable, and financially sound? You don't (even though you are sure that *you* are right). If there are decisions that each of you feels strongly about, then the best course of action is to ask an expert to weigh in. In matters of childcare, ask your pediatrician. If you can't resolve a money question, get a financial planner, banker, or accountant involved. You may find that your spiritual leader can help you resolve issues ranging from child rearing to in-laws. Marriage therapists can also be helpful, particularly if they are focused on helping you define specific problems and helping you learn ways to communicate about them.

It's important to find the right therapist for your relationship, as I've discussed in chapter 4. Poorly trained therapists, or therapists who focus on individuals' (rather than couples') needs, often look at relationship problems as evidence that you would be better off alone. Such advice is not marriage-friendly at all. Studies show that leaving an unhappy marriage does not make people happier unless they are victims of domestic violence. Most of those therapists aren't aware of the many studies showing that people who stay married live longer, richer, and healthier lives than those who divorce. Many therapists are trained to be neutral, but I think it's to your advantage to see therapists who identify themselves as supporting your mutual decision to stay married.

Therapeutic neutrality also conveys the illusion that all points of view are equal. That's ridiculous. If Jack and his wife were to see a therapist, for example, then in my opinion the therapist ought to say, "Mrs. Jack, your expectations are unreasonable. Change your tune."

✤ A MODEL OF MARITAL IDEALS

At the beginning of the last chapter, Amber looks at her affair as a "wake-up call." What about you? Here it is, do or die time. What will you do to change the direction of your marriage? Throughout this chapter, I have asked you to focus on your behaviors and attitude as a way to have the best possible relationship. But you may be concerned that if you take my advice, you will be the only one doing all the work. There's method in my madness. Ideally your partner will read each word of this book and take it to heart as profoundly as you have. But even if he or she hasn't, your ability to improve your marriage can have a powerful impact on your marital happiness.

When your partner begins to see the changes in you and the ways that you are making your relationship a place of comfort, understanding, and positivity, it dramatically lowers the tension in the household and permits him or her to offer some of that marriage-building behavior right back at you. It's a good formula for increasing marital satisfaction, reducing the risk for affairs in the future, and building a lifetime of happiness. You've been through enough; it's what you deserve.

Epilogue

Every writer has a bias. If a writer wants to convince you that windmills are good for the environment, he or she can cite ample evidence to support this view. A different writer can cite evidence to support a strong case *against* windmills. So when you read a book that purports to tell you the "truth" about a subject, it's best to know the bias of the author.

I write about relationships and family. As you will have figured out by reading this book, I have biases of my own. Here they are:

- I have great admiration and respect for the institution of marriage.
- Affairs are the single most destructive act that a marriage must endure.
- Staying married isn't easy, even without affairs, but with proper skills, people can find happiness spending their lives with one partner.

This book includes examples of people who have dealt with affairs but who have learned, either through their own trial and error or with professional guidance, how to get themselves back on track. In chapter 10, we read about a woman who, in the presence of an unrepentant and unrelentingly cheating husband, decides to divorce, and finds happiness two years later. I struggled about whether to include this story, since I have a promarriage bias and did not want my readers to conclude that the answer to infidelity is to divorce and seek happiness elsewhere. Yet I must bow to the reality that the unfaithful partner is sometimes so far beyond repair or the degree of pain felt by the faithful partner is so deep, that there is no realistic expectation of reconciliation.

The secret to surviving infidelity can be summed up with one word: trust. I wrote this book with trust-building in mind. It would be easy to label anyone who has had an affair as having a serious character flaw or as being worthy of contempt. Yet I hope that my discussion of how affairs happen can help people see that even decent, otherwise trustworthy people can stray from their marital vows under the right conditions. Knowing what circumstances can lead to an affair is your best protection against having affairs.

At one point or another you and your partner must open up to each other and talk about the affair. Almost all of these conversations start with minimization, rationalization, even out-and-out lies on the part of the spouse who had an affair, but they don't have to end up that way. Moving forward means facing the facts of what the unfaithful partner has done, ending contact with the affair mate, and making open disclosures about the events of the affair. This process also requires learning how to help each other understand the intensity of feelings that come before, during, and at the end of an extramarital relationship.

Following the chapters on disclosure, I wrote about apology and forgiveness, because these acts are the real turning points for most marriages. It's not easy to say "I'm sorry," but it's a must. For individuals who are deeply hurt by an affair, granting forgiveness also takes strength. When people put aside their pain and grant love in return, it generates a grace that infuses a marriage and propels it forward.

But love and grace aren't enough to keep a marriage strong, just as being madly infatuated with each other when you first met has not kept your relationship free from affairs. Almost every couple believes that they know what skills they need to make marriage work from the moment they get engaged. Very few actually have those skills. In a time when only about half of American adults have been raised by both their parents, there aren't many role models left for good marriage. Combine that with the media's perpetual distortion of what marriage is supposed to look like, and it becomes challenging for couples to find their way to a natural rhythm of marital happiness. That's why in the last three chapters of the book we worked to form more realistic expectations for your marriage.

Most of the people I counsel for marital help have attitudes that fall into one of two categories: either they believe that the purpose of marriage is for their partner to make them happy or they wish to make their partner happy by following the golden rule: "Treat other people as we would wish to be treated ourselves." As I suggest in chapter 11, neither of these approaches is likely to lead to a mutually happy marriage. Rather, I advocate the platinum rule: "Treat people as they wish to be treated." What a difference from the golden rule! When people genuinely take an interest in what makes their mates tick and nurture those passions, their mate notices. When a mate feels loved, more often than not he or she gives love in return.

If I have one other bias, it's that I'm optimistic. I believe that people generally mean well, and even when they hurt others, it's not usually out of spite or with malicious intent. I reveal this bias because it's easy to look at a book that offers to help you get past your affair and say, "Scott has no idea how hard this is for me. Otherwise he wouldn't be trying so hard to help me find a way to make my marriage work." Let me just say that my efforts to cheer you on toward a strong marriage do not reflect ignorance on my part. I have seen firsthand the devastation that an affair leaves in its wake. But the fact that you have been through such a difficult time does not prove to me that there is no hope for your marriage. Many people, like Amber, look at the events of an affair as a wake-up call, both an opportunity to learn about themselves and a chance to learn about their marriage. The process of dealing with affairs has helped people reach out to friends, family members, and spiritual advisors in ways that have improved their connection with the community. Ironically, some people have told me their partner's affair led to a stronger relationship that is more secure than ever before.

It is my hope that this book has helped you get to that place. But I also know that one book will neither answer all your questions nor solve all your problems. If you have found this book helpful, then I encourage you to read it again, because you will surely have missed some things the first time around. I hope you have a chance to build up your relationship with either a marriage education class or with other books designed to help your marriage.

I wish to end this book with a note of tremendous respect for you, the reader. Whether you had an affair and are now looking for ways to reconnect or you have a partner who strayed from the marriage and you wish to rebuild, you *chose* to read this book. I have asked you to take a pretty hard look at yourself. I have challenged you to find ways to heal despite your pain. And I have asked you to learn ways to have a healthy, happy marriage. You've taken on that challenge. Thank you. It's an honor to be part of your life and your future successes.

Notes

Chapter 2. What's Emotion Got to Do with It?

p. 10, *emotional bond with his paramour*: D. M. Buss, R. J. Larsen, D. Westen, and J. Semmelroth, Sex differences in jealousy: Evolution, physiology, and psychology, *Psychological Science* 3 (1992): 251–55.

p. 22, *Simply by looking at pictures of eyes*: Simon Baron-Cohen, *The Essential Difference: Male and Female Brains and the Truth about Autism* (New York: Basic Books, 2004).

p. 22, *But close examination of dating rituals shows the opposite*: M. Moore, Courtship signaling and adolescents: "Girls just wanna have fun?" *Journal of Sex Research* 32, no. 4 (1995): 319.

p. 25, Laurie Puhn, *Fight Less, Love More: 5-Minute Conversations to Change Your Relationship without Blowing Up or Giving In* (Emmaus, PA: Rodale Press, 2010).

Chapter 3. What the Numbers Tell Us

p. 42, *about 1.5 percent of people will have an affair for each year of marriage*: A. Blow and K. Hartnett, Infidelity in committed relationships. II: A substantive review, *Journal of Marital and Family Therapy* 31, no. 2 (2005): 217-33.

p. 42, *have the highest rates of infidelity over a lifetime:* Edward Laumann et al. *The Social Organization of Sexuality and Sexual Practices in the United* States (Chicago: University of Chicago Press, 1994).

p. 43, *70 percent of American women . . . broken their marriage vows at least once*: Shere Hite, *The Hite Report: A Nationwide Study of Female Sexuality* (New York: Random House, 1987).

Chapter 4. Why People Cheat

p. 46, *a 24 percent increase in sexual activity*: A. J. Wilcox et al., On the frequency of intercourse around ovulation: Evidence of biological influences, *Human Reproduction* 19, no. 7 (2004): 1539–43.

p. 47, *often quoted as saying "Love is a dirty trick"*: W. Somerset Maugham, *A Writer's Notebook* (1946) first general edition by Country Life Press (1949), 38.

p. 54, *this human form had enough power to overwhelm the gods*: Plato, "The Symposium," in *The Dialogues,* vol. 2, translated with comment by R. E. Allen (New Haven, CT: Yale University Press, 1991).

p. 56, *they are willing to give out more money to strangers*: M. Kosfeld, M. Heinrichs, P. J. Zak, U. Fischbacher, and E. Fehr, Oxytocin increases trust in humans, *Nature* 435, 7042 (June 2005): 673–76.

p. 57, *the average man will have more sexual partners than the average woman*: Cheryl D. Fryar et al., Drug use and sexual behaviors reported by adults: United States, 1999-2002, *Advance Data From Vital and Health Statistics* 384 (June 28, 2007): 1250.

p. 59, *tend to prefer women based on body shapes*: S. W. Gangestad et al., Changes in women's mate preferences across the ovulatory cycle, *Journal of Personality and Social Psychology* 92, no. 1 (2007): 151–63.

p. 59, *women seek sex for the purposes of emotional closeness*: Daniel D. Sewell, Sexuality, aging and dementia, *Audio-Digest Psychiatry* 36, no. 15 (August 7, 2007). www.cme-ce-summaries.com/psychiatry/ps3615.html.

p. 74, *brain scans of long-married couples who are deeply in love*: B. Acevedo et al., Neural correlates of long-term intense romantic love, *Social Cognitive and Affective Neuroscience* 7, no. 2 (2012): 145-59.

p. 74, *have a surge in their dopamine*: L. A. Sell et al., Activation of reward circuitry in human opiate addicts, *European Journal of Neuroscience* 11, no. 3 (March 1999): 1042–48.

p. 75, *gambling addicts when they are shown a deck of cards*: C. Bergh et al., Altered dopamine function in pathological gambling, *Psychological Medicine* 27 (1997): 473–75.

p. 78, *addictive behaviors in their late teens and early twenties*: B. F. Grant and D. A. Dawson, Introduction to the National Epidemiologic Survey on alcohol and related conditions, *Alcohol Research and Health* 29, no. 2 (2006). http://pubs. niaaa.nih.gov/publications/arh29-2/74-78.pdf.

p. 86, *those who have an identical sibling who strays*: A. D. Fisher, Psychobiological correlates of extramarital affairs and differences between stable and occasional infidelity among men with sexual dysfunctions, *The Journal of Sexual Medicine* 6, no. 3 (March 2009): 866–75. L. F. Cherkas et al. Genetic influences on female infidelity and number of sexual partners in humans: A linkage and association study of the role of the vasopressin receptor gene (AVPR1A), *Twin Research* 7, no. 6 (2004): 649–58.

Chapter 5. Giving the NOD to an Affair

p. 88, *thirteen women were confirmed as objects of Tiger's philandering*: Rodney Page, A year later, Tiger regroups. *Tampa Bay Times,* November 26, 2010. www. tampabay.com/sports/golf/a-year-later-tiger-regroups/1136407.

p. 94, *too many choices leave people feeling*: Barry Schwartz, *The Paradox of Choice: Why More Is Less* (New York: Ecco, 2004).

p. 100, *article about women and infidelity*: Mike Torchia, Confessions of a personal trainer, *Newsweek*, July 12, 2004.

p. 105, *men (but not women) may end up making more short-sighted decisions*: Jonah Lehrer, *How We Decide* (New York: Houghton Mifflin, 2009).

p. 106, *better than others at finding ways to resist impulses*: Yuichi Shoda, Walter Mischel, and Philip K. Peake, Predicting adolescent cognitive and self-regulatory competencies from preschool delay of gratification: Identifying diagnostic conditions. *Developmental Psychology* 26, no. 6 (1990): 978–86.

Chapter 6. Affair Exposed, Now What?

p. 143, *most helpful part of their recovery was the truthful revelation*: Peggy Vaughan, Extramarital Affairs Resource Center, www.DearPeggy.com.

Chapter 7. Getting to the Heart of the Matter

p. 159, *holding the cheating husband responsible for his actions*: Review of M. Gary Neuman, *The Truth about Cheating: Why Men Stray and What You Can Do to Prevent It* (Hoboken, NJ: Wiley, 2008) in *Publishers' Weekly,* http://www.publishersweekly.com/978-0-470-11463-6.

Chapter 8. Forgiveness

p. 184, *more or less reduced to saying some variant of "I'm sorry"*: Erving Goffman, *Relations in Public: Microstudies of the Public Order* (New York: Basic, 1971), 117.

p. 188, *Women are more likely to perceive things*: Karina Schumann and Michael Ross, Why women apologize more than men: Gender differences in thresholds for perceiving offensive behavior, *Psychological Science* 21, no. 11 (November 2010): 1649-55.

p. 193, *Forgiveness welcomes the wrongdoer back*: R. Enright and G. Reed, A definition of forgiveness, *Meet the International Forgiveness Institute Newsletter* (Madison, WI: International Forgiveness Institute), 1997.

p. 198, *offering an apology can lower your levels of anxiety and stress*: http://www.mayoclinic.com/health/forgiveness/MH00131

Chapter 9. What to Expect When You're Expecting (a Happy Marriage)

p. 205, *feeling of dissatisfaction with herself*: Leo Tolstoy, *Anna Karenina* (New York: Penguin Classics, 2004).

p. 211, Lori Gottlieb, *Marry Him: The Case for Settling for Mr. Good Enough* (New York: Dutton Adult, 2010).

p. 218, *if wives want a particular present from their husbands*: Scott Haltzman, *The Secrets of Happily Married Women: How To Get More Out of Your Relationship by Doing Less* (San Francisco: Jossey-Bass, 2008).

p. 219, *take the initiative for remembering their wives' special days*: Scott Haltzman, *The Secrets of Happily Married Men: Eight Ways to Win Your Wife's Heart Forever* (San Francisco: Jossey-Bass, 2006).

p. 221, *the swift wings of my desire would shatter against the iron gates of the impossible*: Stephen Crane, *The Red Badge of Courage* (New York: Airmont, 1962), 119.

p. 224, *we give five times more significance to negative interactions*: John M. Gottman and Nan Silver, *The Seven Principles for Making Marriage Work* (New York: Crown, 1999).

Chapter 10. Ready to Rebuild?

p. 231, *estimate that over half or more*: S. Parnass, The impact of extramarital relationships on the continuation of marriages, *Journal of Sex and Marital Therapy* 21 (1995): 100–115.

p. 233, *By the early 1980s that number skyrocketed to 50 percent*: Vital Statistics of the United States 1950 and 1980, http://www.cdc.gov/nchs/data/vsus/mgdv80_3.pdf and http://www.cdc.gov/nchs/data/vsus/VSUS_1950_2.pdf.

p. 235, Thornton Wilder, *The Skin of Our Teeth* (New York: Perennial Classics, 2003), 79 (original work published 1943).

Chapter 11. Building a Better Marriage

p. 252, *gender differences when it comes to communication*: Simon Baron-Cohen, *The Essential Difference: Male and Female Brains and the Truth about Autism* (New York: Basic Books, 2004).

p. 253, Deborah Tannen, *You Just Don't Understand: Men and Women in Conversation* (New York: Morrow, 2001).

p. 259, *when you get flooded with emotions*: John M. Gottman and Nan Silver, *The Seven Principles for Making Marriage Work* (New York: Crown, 1999).

p. 262, Gary Chapman, *The Five Love Languages: The Secret to Love That Lasts* (Chicago: Northfield Publishing, 2009).

p. 265, Amy Sutherland, *What Shamu Taught Me about Life, Love, and Marriage: Lessons for People from Animals and Their Trainers* (New York: Random House, 2009).

p. 268, *Researchers at State University of New York*: Greg Strong and Arthur Aron, The effect of shared participation in novel and challenging activities on experienced relationship quality: Is it mediated by high positive affect? In Kathleen D. Vohs & Eli J. Finkel (Eds.), *Self and Relationships: Connecting Intrapersonal and Interpersonal Processes* (New York: Guilford, 2006), 342–59.

p. 270, Esther Perel, *Mating in Captivity: Unlocking Erotic Intelligence* (New York: Harper Perennial, 2007).

p. 271, *75 percent of men describe themselves as having a higher sex drive than their wives*: Scott Haltzman, Correlates of sexual desire in married men [Poster], Coalition for Marriage, Family and Couples Education Annual Meeting, Reno, NV, June 24-27, 2003.

p. 273, *starting some foreplay with an attractive mate*: R. Basson, Sexual desire and arousal disorders in women, *New England Journal of Medicine* 354 (2006): 1497-1506.

p. 276, *marriage helps protect people against a host of . . . problems*: Linda Waite and Maggie Gallagher, *A Case for Marriage: Why Married People Are Happier, Healthier, and Better Off Financially* (New York: Broadway, 2001).

p. 279, *leaving an unhappy marriage does not make people happier*: Linda Waite and Maggie Gallagher, *A Case for Marriage: Why Married People Are Happier, Healthier, and Better Off Financially* (New York: Broadway, 2001), and Linda Waite et al., Does divorce make people happy? Findings from a study of unhappy marriages. Institute for American Values report, 2002.

Epilogue

p. 283, *only about half of American adults have been raised by both their parents*: David T. Ellwood and Christopher Jencks, *The Spread of Single-Parent Families in the United States since 1960* (February 26, 2004). John F. Kennedy School of Government Working Paper No. RWP04-008, Harvard University. Available at SSRN: http://ssrn.com/abstract=517662 or http://dx.doi.org/10.2139/ssrn.517662.

About the Author

SCOTT HALTZMAN, M.D., is a distinguished fellow of the American Psychiatric Association and former clinical assistant professor of psychiatry at Brown University. He is the author of *The Secrets of Happily Married Men*, *The Secrets of Happily Married Women*, and *The Secrets of Happy Families*. You can reach him at Facebook.com/ScottHaltzman or at DrHaltzman@secretsofmarriedmen.com.

Index